# THE MENSTRUAL CYCLE

KATHARINA
DALTON, M.D.

# The
# Menstrual
# Cycle

 PANTHEON BOOKS · A Division of
Random House, New York

618
DAm

# Contents

# Foreword

The success of women who share with men the top posts of the professions, industry, commerce and politics, gives credence to the claims for equality of the sexes. Apart from the obvious sex differences, the vital organs of the body are identical and operate in the same way, but the woman has an important difference associated with the reproductive function. It is this difference that affects her personality and behavior pattern. Woman's reproductive process requires a complicated system of chemical controls which would seem to be unique and is altogether different from that found in the male. This is probably why so little has been known about the commonest disease in the world, the premenstrual syndrome.

For more than twenty years, as husband and ghost-writer, I have shared with Dr. Katharina Dalton the task of piecing together the results of her clinical observations of menstruation in several thousands of women, revealing the kaleidoscopic effects of the menstrual cycle on their lives. These findings she has set down in this book so that all who read it may understand the extent to which the cyclical changes in the levels of a woman's hormones are responsible for her unpredictable changes of personality. The reader will begin to realize that there is a biological basis for much that has been written, or said, about the whims and vagaries of women.

The old cliché, "It's a woman's privilege to change her mind," calls for an even greater tolerance than before now that it is realized that every woman is at the mercy of the constantly recurring ebb and flow of her hormones.

TOM E. DALTON

*March 1968*

# Preface

There are a number of variations in the patterns of menstruation which come within the bounds of normality, but have attendant discomfort and suffering, both physical and mental. These variations are rarely to be found in any textbook but have a considerable sociological impact on society: they and their consequences are the subject of this book. It is my hope that by opening up this subject to a wider audience I may induce women to appreciate that there is an answer to much of today's unnecessary suffering; that men may gain a sympathetic understanding of the problems of the opposite sex; and that my medical colleagues may appreciate how much work remains to be done to alleviate the sufferings of women in the sphere of normal menstruation.

In my first paper on the premenstrual syndrome, given at the Royal Society of Medicine in 1954, I remarked that this work "opened up a new vista of Medicine." At that time I was not aware that the bounds of that vista were so limitless. Research into the premenstrual syndrome has revealed the extent to which the cyclical changes of the levels of a woman's hormones are responsible for her personality changes. The symptoms caused by the menstrual changes are relevant to every medical speciality, are of extraordinary diversity and are found in women the world over.

Much of the work has been previously published in the medical press and I express my thanks to the Editors of the *British Medical Journal, Proceedings of the Royal Society of Medicine, Journal of the Royal College of General Practitioners,* Heinemann Medical Books Ltd., the *British Journal of Psychiatry,* the *Lancet* and the *British Journal of Ophthalmology* for permission to reprint figures from their publications. A full list of publications is contained on pages 143–44 for the more serious student.

Finally, thanks to my husband, who has taken my incoherent notes and made them intelligible for all.

KATHARINA DALTON

*March 1968*

# THE MENSTRUAL CYCLE

# 1

# Being a Woman

When a mother is delivered of her baby there is barely time to inform her that all is over and a fine baby is lustily announcing its arrival in the world, when she asks, "Is it a boy or a girl?" There follows a hasty look at the genitals before the nurse or doctor gives the answer. It is the difference of the sex organs which indicates the future role the baby is to play in society.

Should it be a girl, then the essential biological role of childbearing will be hers. To fulfill this function she is provided with special anatomical organs which develop as she reaches puberty into a most efficient, though complicated, system of monthly preparation for childbearing. Each month a lining is built up within the womb and if no pregnancy occurs it is broken down again and removed in the flow of blood we know as menstruation.

Menstruation describes the physiological process which occurs with monthly regularity for approximately thirty years of a woman's life. It is a word rarely heard outside medical circles. It is used occasionally by women and although its meaning is fully understood by secondary-school children, it is a word seldom used by men. Instead euphemisms are used, as if it were blasphemous, immoral or indecent to use the correct word: some are dull and factual like "monthlies" or "periods"; some are descriptive like "the curse," "unwell," "the blues," or "the wrong day of the month"; others conjure up ideas of familiarity with an old friend, like "Charlie" or "Archie." A French nun refers to menstruation as "The British have landed," which she maintains goes back to the years before the Normandy invasion. Although its origin is forgotten, it is similar to "The Redcoats are Coming," which is still occasionally heard in England today.

At a time when sex is so openly discussed, this blinkered attitude to menstruation is utterly Victorian. Only recently has the subject been considered to be respectable enough to mention in the press or radio. In fact, before any article on the subject appears in a woman's magazine a special consultation with the editor is called for. When a radio or television talk on the subject is to be given, the announcer is likely to warn listeners of the precise time the talk will take, in case there are any who feel the subject is unsuitable for youngsters.

Such an ostrich-like attitude to a subject that involves all mankind is indeed strange. Women have to be prepared to meet the arrival of menstruation each month, and the average woman will have to cope with it some 400 times in her life—so too will men for, whether they are fathers, husbands or sons, their contact with women, at work, at home and at play, will extend throughout their lives.

One would expect that the natural and essential process of menstruation would be painless like other physiological functions of the body such as respiration or digestion, yet rarely does a woman go through life without an occasional painful or troublesome menstruation. When expectant mothers are taught about early labor pains, it is suggested that the first contractions are similar in sensation and position to period pains. If the women are then asked if they would recognize such pains, their reactions show that these are a familiar experience.

These two complementary physiological processes of menstruation and childbirth, although natural functions of human reproduction, are not without their problems. Few people will claim that natural childbirth is entirely free from pain, and menstruation also has its discomforts. There is no justification for the claim that it is our higher civilization that is responsible, when in the Bible is written, "Be in pain and labour to bring forth, O daughter of Zion, like a woman in travail" (Micah 4: 10). Nor can the stresses of modern life be blamed for the tensions attendant upon menstruation; Hippocrates recognized their existence and deduced that the many and varied symptoms were due to the "agitated blood of the womb seeking a way of escape from the body."

The vague sensations preceding the commencement of menstruation can be useful, for to be forewarned removes the fear of being caught unprepared. Nature has endowed the human being with special sensations warning that the bladder is full or the bowels loaded. The sensations are strong enough to awaken the sleeper from the deepest slumbers, so avoiding wetting the bed. In the early days of hormone treatment for menstrual disorders, several women were so completely relieved of the warning sensations of menstruation that they complained bitterly of having ruined their best dresses or having some most embarrassing moments.

The blind are particularly vulnerable in this respect and have a very natural fear that they may leave some tell-tale sign of menstruation on their clothes, of which they themselves are unaware. There was one blind spinster who pleaded for her womb to be removed because menstruation was so free from pain or discomfort that she was never able to appreciate the moment of onset.

But it is a far cry from the complete absence of warning signals of imminent menstruation to the incapacitating pains or the prostration that can regularly interrupt a woman's life. Any recurrent menstrual symptoms which regularly require more than one aspirin for relief, produce a dislocation of a woman's life or interrupt the domestic harmony are deserving of effective medical care.

In October 1965 the magazine *Which?*\* inserted a small notice asking for women volunteers to participate in a scheme for the testing of a product for the relief of period pains, which could be bought over the drugstore counter. Within a short time more than 600 replies had been received. The readers were asked to complete a four-page legal-size form giving personal particulars. Undaunted, almost all completed and returned their forms promptly. The replies were from the middle-class readership and included all ages from fifteen to fifty-five years. The comments accompanying some of the forms should make any diligent doctor blush, for these women wrote of the lack of sympathy and understanding they had received from male doctors. One woman wrote that the doctor had said, "You can't expect the National Health Service to deal with this sort of pain." Another commented, "I was told it would go when I had a child, I've now got two children, how many more do I need?" Nor could it be said that the replies came from those who had failed to respond to medical treatment; two thirds of these women had borne their sufferings without seeking medical advice.

Anesthetics to relieve the pangs of childbirth have been followed, a century later, by the advent of synthetic hormones to relieve the problems of menstruation. It

---

\* The British magazine *Which?* is similar to the American *Consumer Reports.*

took a long time for the use of analgesics in childbirth, introduced in the Victorian era, to be universally accepted. One hopes that the universal recognition and treatment of menstrual discomforts will not take as long.

# 2

# Body Chemistry

Every year, medical science provides us with a greater understanding of the human body and the ways in which it functions. "Body Chemistry" is a phrase that is increasingly used to describe the physiological processes and, indeed, the human body can be likened to a chemical factory with its production centers and its distribution centers.

It is a chemical factory producing a multiplicity of chemicals that are constantly required to keep the many systems of the body functioning properly. In this chapter we are concerned with the production and distribution centers of the chemicals which affect menstruation. It is important to keep in mind that our knowledge of this body chemistry is far from complete, and new information is being added each year. Nevertheless, enough is known to enable us to understand what is basically happening in menstruation and childbirth. Before going into the chemistry, an understanding of the physical process will be helpful.

At any time after her tenth birthday a girl may find signs of a slight discharge from the vagina; gradually this discharge will become red in color and increase in quantity and frequency until the monthly bleeding of menstruation is established. Already the changes of puberty will have been noticed: hair will be growing in the armpits and in the pubic region, and the breasts will have begun to develop. The discharge is the first outward sign that the womb is learning to shed that lining which, from now onwards for the next thirty to forty years, will be formed afresh each month in preparation for the function of childbearing.

In these early months of menstruation no egg cells are released, since the lining of the womb, which is called the *endometrium,* is not yet ready to perform its seedbed function. After a couple of years of menstruation the endometrium is ready and the ovaries take up their task of releasing an ovum or egg cell every month with near clockwork regularity for the next thirty or forty years. This cycle of operations commences at the time the endometrium is being shed at menstruation. In one of the ovaries, which contain thousands of egg cells that have been there since before the girl was born, one of those egg cells is enlarging in preparation for its launching from the wall of the ovary about fourteen days after the beginning of menstruation. Once released from the ovary the egg cell is propelled down the Fallopian tube and into the womb. If no fertilization occurs the egg cell will eventually pass out of the neck of the womb. It is then that the endometrium distintegrates and is flushed out of the womb by the flow of menstrual blood. By this time one of the ovaries is again ripening another egg cell to repeat the process which is the woman's prime biological purpose of life.

The only time, during childbearing years, that this cycle is interrupted is when pregnancy occurs. That can only happen if one of the male sperms, entering through the neck of the womb, finds the egg cell and fertilizes it. When this occurs the fertilized egg cell becomes embedded in the new endometrium. The endometrium gradually gets thicker and the neck of the womb closes, thus ensuring that the pregnancy continues. Meanwhile the egg-laying cycle, including menstruation, is suspended for the duration of the pregnancy. After the baby has been born there is usually a lapse of three to nine months before the egg-laying cycle is resumed; this allows for the breast feeding of the new-born child.

Although this account of the physical processes of menstruation has been presented as though everything happens automatically, it is as well to appreciate that nothing ever happens automatically in the human body; everything that occurs does so in response to some stimulation or other. The sequence of events in the menstrual cycle is governed by physiological processes taking place in other parts of the body. A brief outline of these processes follows.

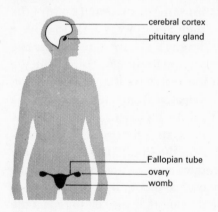

Figure 1. Control of menstruation

The network of nerves sends stimuli from all over the human body to the *cerebral cortex* located in the brain. The cerebral cortex sorts the messages, sending the relevant impulses to the control center of menstruation located in the *hypothalamus,* which is situated at the base of the brain. This in turn feeds information to the *pituitary gland,* which influences the different production centers of the menstrual system (Figure 1). The "menstrual clock" is situated at the base of the brain and regulates the timing of the menstrual cycle to about twenty-eight days. The hypothalamus is affected by the stresses of daily life and also by emotional causes. A later chapter shows how emotions can play an important part in altering the timing of the menstrual clock.

The pituitary gland is the control center of the *endocrine system* and it sends its orders to the various production centers by special chemical messengers called *hormones*. It has often been called the "Leader of the Endocrine Orchestra" because of the way its hormones control the other endocrine glands. In particular it sends hormones to the breasts to prepare for lactation, and to the ovaries to ripen the egg cells. Different hormones leave the pituitary at different times of the menstrual cycle for different tasks.

The physiological pattern of menstruation begins as the menstrual flow commences, with one of the pituitary hormones passing in the bloodstream to stimulate the ripening of one of the thousands of egg cells. Normally only one egg cell in one of the ovaries ripens each month. The minute cell comes gradually to the surface of the ovary, where it forms a small blister or *follicle*. At the same time the ovary is producing a hormone, called *estrogen,* which flows in the bloodstream to the endometrium to prepare it for the reception of the egg cell. About fourteen days after the commencement of menstruation, *ovulation* occurs; this means that the ripened egg cell bursts from the follicle in the wall of the ovary, starting on its journey down the Fallopian tube to the womb. At ovulation messages are sent back to the pituitary gland, which reacts by sending other hormones to the ovary. These stimulate the empty follicle, which becomes filled with specialized cells capable of forming a new production center for another ovarian hormone, called *progesterone*. This new hormone, progesterone, is passed in the blood to the endometrium, where it stimulates the proliferation of the endometrial cells so that the fertilized egg may have a moist and receptive surface into which it can easily become embedded.

As explained earlier, pregnancy will occur only if one of the male sperms that reach the inner surface of the womb fertilizes the egg cell. If this occurs the fertilized egg cell becomes embedded in the prepared endometrium and immediately hormonal messages are sent back to the pituitary with the information that pregnancy has occurred and that a different set of hormones will be required to maintain the pregnancy. If the egg cell is not fertilized it is carried out through the neck of the womb with the endometrial lining which, being no longer required, disintegrates and flows out in the blood that is washing it away and cleaning the cavity. Thus menstruation represents a failed pregnancy, and may be seen as a monthly spring-cleaning in preparation for the next potential pregnancy.

When pregnancy does not occur the menstrual cycle repeats itself, and even while menstruation is proceeding another egg cell in one of the ovaries is ripening in readiness for its release at ovulation. The entire process is regulated by the pituitary hormones and the two ovarian hormones, estrogen and progesterone. There is not a day in a woman's life when she is not subject to the ebb and flow of these hormones.

All the endocrine glands in the body are interrelated and a disturbance in one of them, for example the *thyroid gland,* can result in a change of the normal menstrual rhythm. Probably the most important hormones, and yet the least understood, are those secreted by the two *adrenal glands*. The adrenals are small triangular glands, one situated above each kidney. The central part of the adrenals produce adrenaline, which is concerned with the personal defense mechanisms of fight, flight and fear. The outside part produces numerous vital hormones, known as *corticosteroids,* which control the body's water and salt regulation, the sugar metabolism, the natural defense mechanisms against disease, injury and stress, and are also partially responsible for the secondary sex characteristics. These corticosteroids are formed by some forty different chemical reactions taking place within the adrenals. The most significant finding appears to be that progesterone is the base out of which all the other adrenal corticosteroids are formed. So, even if the ovarian production of progesterone is stopped by the removal of the ovaries, there will still be progesterone present in the adrenal glands. Most of this progesterone is immediately converted into the other corticosteroids, such as aldosterone, corticosterone and cortisol. Aldosterone is the hormone with the task of regulating the water and salt content of the body. This means that excess aldosterone or deficient aldosterone-antagonist causes water retention.

From all this it is easy to appreciate the importance of the body chemistry. The great question that arises is deciding what is normal menstruation for any one individual.

# 3

# Normal Menstruation

Women may experience an infinite variety of types of menstruation, all of which can be quite normal.

Mention has already been made of the reluctance even today to use the word menstruation. Undoubtedly, in the past, the subject has been considered unmentionable; this may well be one reason for the lack of general knowledge about this essential function of a woman's life, and a contributory factor to the endless "old wives' tales" that abound.

It is not surprising that every woman considers that her own particular menstrual pattern is normal until she finds that someone else has a very different one. Then she may, indeed, suddenly fear that she is abnormal. But normality in the menstrual pattern covers an extremely wide field, and it does not matter at all which pattern any woman has.

Variation occurs in the length of the cycle, the duration of loss, the amount and type of blood lost each month. So too there are other physical variations in women such as weight, height, and bust, waist and hip measurements. How does one decide what is normal?

The average interval between the beginning of one menstruation and the next is twenty-eight days, and this is known as the "menstrual cycle," for during this time the changes in the womb complete one cycle before starting to repeat the process. This figure of twenty-eight days only represents the average and not the normal.

When a woman says that her cycle is twenty-eight days, she probably means that it averages out at that figure taken over a period of time, but month by month the actual intervals may be 26–30–26–27–31–28–29 days. Anyone with a cycle of twenty-eight days would find that it always started on the same day of the week. Women on the Pill or being treated with hormones may achieve this precise twenty-eight-day cycle, but it is rare to find anyone not taking hormones with a precisely regular twenty-eight-day cycle. There is a story of a mid-European principality where a woman could claim the title of "Menstrual Princess" and receive a state pension if her menstrual cycle was a precisely regular twenty-eight days. This, of course, was for a perfectly natural cycle and not for one falsely created by hormone treatment. Certainly, in England today, there would be very few aspirants to this title.

In fact one finds perfectly normal, healthy women with cycles varying between twenty and thirty-six days. A cycle of twenty-six days may seem long for the woman used to a three-weekly one, whereas another woman whose cycle is usually five weeks may consider twenty-nine days a short cycle. Both have their advantages. The woman with the short cycle does not have to wait so long to know whether or not she is pregnant, while the one with the long cycle has fewer menstruations per year.

Doctors soon learn how to interpret the answers commonly given in reply to the question "How often does menstruation occur?" The answer, "Oh, I'm always regular," is likely to mean a short cycle and that the woman never gets worried about menstruation being delayed. The one who answers, "I'm always late," really means that her cycle exceeds the conventional twenty-eight days.

It is of great value for each woman to work out the normal length of her cycle. There is a surprisingly large number of women who, while marking their dates carefully in their diaries, will mark twenty-eight days ahead to represent the next expected menstruation. In fact the actual cycle will normally be several days more or less than this

| | Jan. | Feb. | Mar. | Apr. | May | Jun. | Jul. | Aug. | Sep. | Oct. | Nov. | Dec. |
|---|---|---|---|---|---|---|---|---|---|---|---|---|
| 1 | | | | | | | | P | | | | |
| 2 | | | | | | | | P | | | | |
| 3 | | | | | | | P | P | | | | |
| 4 | | | | | | | P | | | | | |
| 5 | | | | | | P | P | | | | | |
| 6 | | | | | | P | P | | | | | |
| 7 | | | | | | P | | | | | | |
| 8 | | | | | P | P | | | | | | |
| 9 | | | | | P | | | | | | | |
| 10 | | | | P | P | | | | | | | |
| 11 | | | | P | P | | | | | | | |
| 12 | | | | P | | | | | | | | |
| 13 | | | P | P | | | | | | | | |
| 14 | | P | P | | | | | | | | | |
| 15 | | P | P | | | | | | | | | |
| 16 | | P | P | | | | | | | | | |
| 17 | P | P | | | | | | | | | | |
| 18 | P | | | | | | | | | | | P |
| 19 | P | | | | | | | | | | | P |
| 20 | P | | | | | | | | | | P | P |
| 21 | | | | | | | | | | | P | P |
| 22 | | | | | | | | | | P | P | |
| 23 | | | | | | | | | | P | P | |
| 24 | | | | | | | | | P | P | | |
| 25 | | | | | | | | | P | P | | |
| 26 | | | | | | | | | P | | | |
| 27 | | | | | | | | | P | | | |
| 28 | | | | | | | | P | | | | |
| 29 | | | | | | | | P | | | | |
| 30 | | | | | | | | P | | | | |
| 31 | | | | | | | P | P | | | | |
| Total | | | | | | | | | | | | |

Figure 2. Menstrual chart showing cycle of 28 days and 4 days duration

date. They have the idea so firmly fixed in their minds that it must be twenty-eight days, that they lose sight of the actual length of their personal cycles.

Some women have shorter cycles at certain seasons of the year, often in the warm summer months. Others will notice a short and a longer cycle alternating. Both are within normal limits.

There is really only one way of showing the regularity and duration of menstruation: that is with the use of a menstrual chart (Figure 2).

The information entered on the chart can be seen in a glance; it will show whether the cycle and duration are regular or irregular, short or long. Estimating the ex-

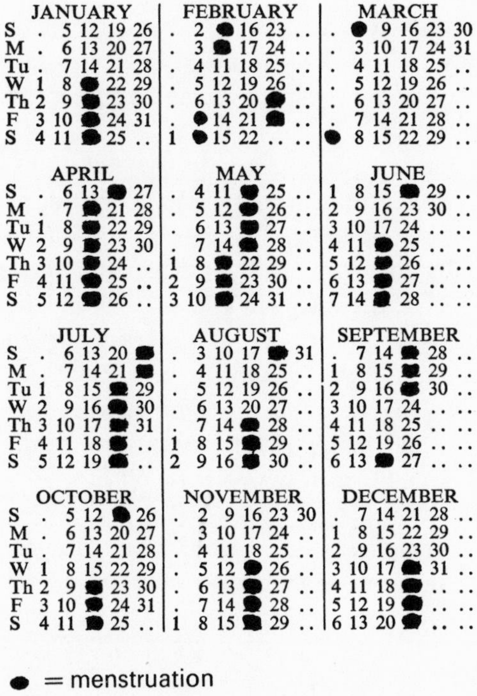

```
       JANUARY      |      FEBRUARY    |       MARCH
S  .  5 12 19 26    |  .  2 ● 16 23 .. |  .  ●  9 16 23 30
M  .  6 13 20 27    |  .  3 ● 17 24 .. |  .  3 10 17 24 31
Tu .  7 14 21 28    |  .  4 11 18 25 . |  .  4 11 18 25 ..
W  1  8 ● 22 29     |  .  5 12 19 26 . |  .  5 12 19 26 ..
Th 2  9 ● 23 30     |  .  6 13 20 ●  . |  .  6 13 20 27 ..
F  3 10 ● 24 31     |  .  ● 14 21 ●  . |  .  7 14 21 28 ..
S  4 11 ● 25 ..     |  1  ● 15 22 ... . |  ●  8 15 22 29 ..

        APRIL       |        MAY       |        JUNE
S  .  6 13 ● 27     |  .  4 11 ● 25 .. | 1  8 15 ● 29 ..
M  .  7 ● 21 28     |  .  5 12 ● 26 .. | 2  9 16 23 30 ..
Tu 1  8 ● 22 29     |  .  6 13 ● 27 .. | 3 10 17 24 . ..
W  2  9 ● 23 30     |  .  7 14 ● 28 .. | 4 11 ● 25 . ..
Th 3 10 ● 24 ..     | 1  8 ● 22 29 ..  | 5 12 ● 26 . ..
F  4 11 ● 25 ..     | 2  9 ● 23 30 ..  | 6 13 ● 27 . ..
S  5 12 ● 26 ..     | 3 10 ● 24 31 ..  | 7 14 ● 28 . ..

        JULY        |       AUGUST     |     SEPTEMBER
S  .  6 13 20 ●     |  .  3 10 17 ● 31 |  .  7 14 ● 28 ..
M  .  7 14 21 ●     |  .  4 11 18 25 .. | 1  8 15 ● 29 ..
Tu 1  8 15 ● 29     |  .  5 12 19 26 .. | 2  9 16 ● 30 ..
W  2  9 16 ● 30     |  .  6 13 20 27 .. | 3 10 17 24 . ..
Th 3 10 17 ● 31     |  .  7 14 ● 28 ..  | 4 11 18 25 . ..
F  4 11 18 ● ..     | 1  8 15 ● 29 ..   | 5 12 19 26 . ..
S  5 12 19 ● ..     | 2  9 16 ● 30 ..   | 6 13 ● 27 . ..

      OCTOBER       |     NOVEMBER     |     DECEMBER
S  .  5 12 ● 26     |  .  2  9 16 23 30 |  .  7 14 21 28 ..
M  .  6 13 20 27    |  .  3 10 17 24 .. | 1  8 15 22 29 ..
Tu .  7 14 21 28    |  .  4 11 18 25 .. | 2  9 16 23 30 ..
W  1  8 15 22 29    |  .  5 12 ● 26 ..  | 3 10 17 ● 31 ..
Th 2  9 ● 23 30     |  .  6 13 ● 27 ..  | 4 11 18 ● . ..
F  3 10 ● 24 31     |  .  7 14 ● 28 ..  | 5 12 19 ● . ..
S  4 11 ● 25 ..     | 1  8 15 ● 29 ..   | 6 13 20 ● . ..
```

● = menstruation

Figure 3. Calendar—compare ease of recognizing menstrual pattern with menstrual chart on Figure 2

pected date of the next menstruation becomes a simple task. Most women use the small calendar at the end of their diary as shown in Figure 3, but such deductions cannot be made without complicated calculations on this type of calendar.

In hospitals these charts are called "frequency charts" and are used to plot the frequency of chronically recurring aches and pains. The charts have other uses as will be seen in later chapters.

The duration of menstruation is also as variable as the length of the cycle. The bleeding may last for a mere two days or may continue for a full seven days. Bleeding may even stop or slow down for a day or two and then begin again. Some women have their heaviest bleeding on the first day and then lose very little, while others start with a slight blood loss which gradually increases after a few days. All these variations are within normal limits of good health (Figure 4).

The actual amount of blood lost may be very slight, barely marking one napkin, or it may be so heavy that it soaks three napkins in one hour. The description of the amount lost is usually only the personal assessment by one who has never seen another woman's loss. It should be realized that only a small quantity of blood is necessary to turn a bucket of water bright red. In the same way, any menstrual blood passing into the toilet bowl will soon make all the water look like blood, but this should never be taken as an assessment of how much blood has been lost.

Even today one occasionally meets women who are terrified that, because their blood loss is so scanty, the blood is accumulating somewhere within them, and that one day it will poison them to death or be lost in one fearful hemorrhage. Others are frightened that in losing too much blood they will bleed to death. They need have no fear for this can never happen during menstruation.

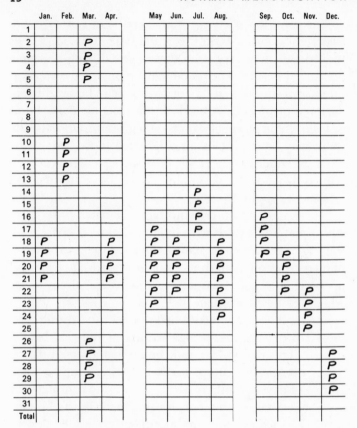

Figure 4. Charts showing variations of the menstrual cycle

Menstrual bleeding is from minute capillaries, which are exposed when the endometrium disintegrates. The capillaries are soon plugged by the formation of blood clots. There are no large blood vessels near the lining of the womb from which serious bleeding can occur.

The amount of blood lost by healthy women, who are on a good diet, is quickly regained. For those who have a tendency to develop anemia it is well worthwhile taking a daily iron tablet to prevent any possibility of anemia occurring.

The infinite variety, so characteristic of normal menstruation, is also seen in the actual type of blood passed; indeed this may vary from day to day during the same menstrual period. The blood may be pink and watery, as often seen on the first day or two. It may be bright red, dark red or practically black. It may include dark shreds or even whole pieces of dark red membrane. Occasionally there may be small clots of bright red blood, but if the clots are larger than a grape, or if their passage is accompanied by pain, this should be regarded as abnormal and treatment sought.

Severe pain or other symptoms associated with menstruation will be dealt with in later chapters. Apart from the vague sensations signaling the approach of the onset of menstruation, pain should not be regarded as a normal or inevitable accompaniment, but as an abnormality which requires treatment.

Earlier it has been mentioned that menstruation represents a physiological spring-cleaning of the womb each month. The analogy can now be carried a stage further. Some housewives complete their spring-cleaning in a couple of days and others take many days to complete the same task. Some use a lot of cleaning materials and others manage to achieve the same results using less. Some will tackle the task more frequently than others. Whichever pattern is used, the home still remains a home and its normal function continues unabated. The same is true of menstruation, for, whatever the menstrual pattern, pregnancy can occur in any one of the variations mentioned in this chapter.

# 4

# Emotions and
# the Menstrual Clock

The value of knowing your own menstrual pattern will become self-evident by the time you have read this chapter, which deals with the way the emotions can affect the normal pattern.

In the second chapter it was shown that the cycle was governed by a menstrual clock located in the base of the brain. It is stimulated by impulses of our conscious thoughts and actions relayed from the cerebral cortex. These stimulations, if of sufficient intensity, effectively alter the normal menstrual cycle. It is a common enough experience for a young girl to find that on the night of that long awaited first big event, whether it is a dance, a theater or a dinner party, her menstruation has commenced.

Of course it is not only the menstrual pattern that is affected by emotional stresses and strains; our other bodily processes are also affected. The exciting news of winning a football pool, or the sudden death of a close relative or a great friend can be the cause of sudden loss of appetite and can prevent normal sleep.

The extent to which emotion can influence the normal menstrual pattern has recently been demonstrated in a girls' boarding school. Ninety-one of the girls, whose ages were between fourteen and seventeen years, were all taking their "O-level" examinations, standard high school examinations, of vital importance and likely to influence their entire future career. Just under half of these girls showed an alteration in their normal menstrual pattern. In many the cycle was lengthened, in some it was shortened, and some missed their menstruation completely. Another important finding was that many more girls than usual were menstruating on the vital days of the examinations. Of the ninety-one candidates, an average of sixteen girls normally menstruated on any one day during the month of May, but during the one week of examinations in June as many as thirty-six girls were menstruating on one day (Figure 5).

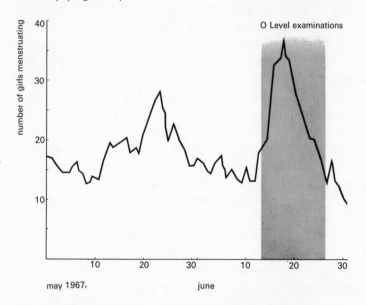

Figure 5. Time of menstruation of examination candidates

Thus, although the menstrual pattern was altered by the same emotional stress, each individual girl had her own variable response to that stress.

No one can go through life entirely without emotional

stresses. Sometimes these are wonderfully exciting experiences like weddings, holidays, parties and financial gains and sometimes they are experiences of the other sort like bereavement, moving to a new house, changing jobs, interviews or examinations. All those stresses are experi-

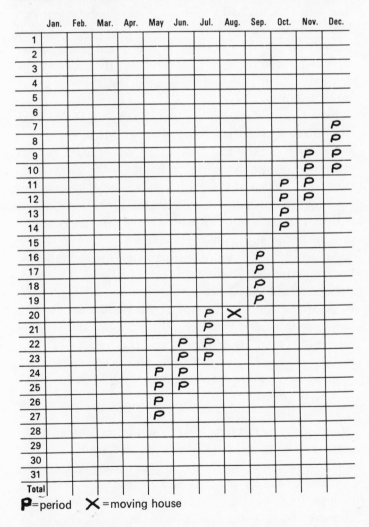

**P**=period  **X**=moving house

Figure 6. Missed menstruation on house-moving day

enced by the cerebral cortex and relayed to our menstrual clock, so affecting the normal menstrual rhythm.

The response to a given stress is variable and individual. Figure 6 shows the chart of a woman, forty-three years of age and mother of two children, who had to move to a new house about half-a-mile away on August twentieth. Her menstruation was due on the day of the move; instead she missed that menstruation entirely, and resumed her normal pattern in September with menstruation on the day that would have been expected had there been no interruption.

Now look at the chart in Figure 7 which is of a woman of similar age, also the mother of two children. She had to move her home from London to the Sussex coast. She became very tense and worried at the planning involved in the move. The effect of all this stress was to give her a prolonged menstruation lasting eighteen days, but the normal pattern was restored without any treatment as she settled down happily in her new home.

An acquaintance who travels about Europe finds that her menstruations always occur in each capital. This emotional effect of travel on the menstrual clock is confirmed by teachers who take groups of schoolchildren abroad. One of their chief difficulties is that far more of their girls menstruate than would have been expected. A girl's first menstruation is likely to begin on such occasions. Several mothers have said to me, "I sent away a girl and a young woman returned."

In much the same way, "depression" has a variable effect on the menstrual clock. When women become depressed their menstruation may become scanty or even absent, and this is especially likely to occur if the weight becomes markedly reduced and the appetite is lost, as happens in a nervous complaint called *anorexia nervosa*. However there are people who, when they become depressed, develop prolonged menstruation. This condition

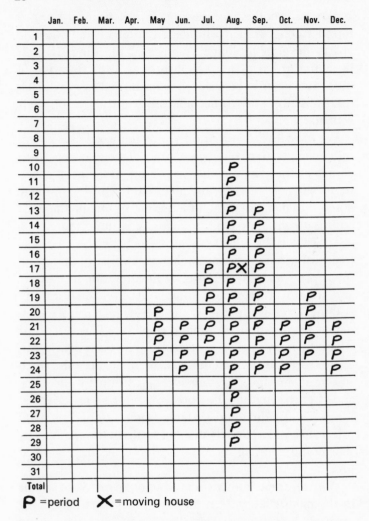

|  | Jan. | Feb. | Mar. | Apr. | May | Jun. | Jul. | Aug. | Sep. | Oct. | Nov. | Dec. |
|---|---|---|---|---|---|---|---|---|---|---|---|---|
| 1 |  |  |  |  |  |  |  |  |  |  |  |  |
| 2 |  |  |  |  |  |  |  |  |  |  |  |  |
| 3 |  |  |  |  |  |  |  |  |  |  |  |  |
| 4 |  |  |  |  |  |  |  |  |  |  |  |  |
| 5 |  |  |  |  |  |  |  |  |  |  |  |  |
| 6 |  |  |  |  |  |  |  |  |  |  |  |  |
| 7 |  |  |  |  |  |  |  |  |  |  |  |  |
| 8 |  |  |  |  |  |  |  |  |  |  |  |  |
| 9 |  |  |  |  |  |  |  |  |  |  |  |  |
| 10 |  |  |  |  |  |  |  | P |  |  |  |  |
| 11 |  |  |  |  |  |  |  | P |  |  |  |  |
| 12 |  |  |  |  |  |  |  | P |  |  |  |  |
| 13 |  |  |  |  |  |  |  | P | P |  |  |  |
| 14 |  |  |  |  |  |  |  | P | P |  |  |  |
| 15 |  |  |  |  |  |  |  | P | P |  |  |  |
| 16 |  |  |  |  |  |  |  | P | P |  |  |  |
| 17 |  |  |  |  |  |  | P | PX | P |  |  |  |
| 18 |  |  |  |  |  |  | P | P | P |  |  |  |
| 19 |  |  |  |  |  |  | P | P | P |  | P |  |
| 20 |  |  |  |  | P |  | P | P | P |  | P |  |
| 21 |  |  |  |  | P | P | P | P | P | P | P | P |
| 22 |  |  |  |  | P | P | P | P | P | P | P | P |
| 23 |  |  |  |  | P | P | P | P | P | P | P | P |
| 24 |  |  |  |  |  | P |  | P | P | P |  | P |
| 25 |  |  |  |  |  |  |  | P |  |  |  |  |
| 26 |  |  |  |  |  |  |  | P |  |  |  |  |
| 27 |  |  |  |  |  |  |  | P |  |  |  |  |
| 28 |  |  |  |  |  |  |  | P |  |  |  |  |
| 29 |  |  |  |  |  |  |  | P |  |  |  |  |
| 30 |  |  |  |  |  |  |  |  |  |  |  |  |
| 31 |  |  |  |  |  |  |  |  |  |  |  |  |
| Total |  |  |  |  |  |  |  |  |  |  |  |  |

**P** = period   **X** = moving house

Figure 7. Prolonged menstruation at the time of house-moving

has been called the "weeping womb." Both these alterations in the menstrual rhythm can be restored to normality by removing the depression with some of the marvel-
lous anti-depressant drugs that are available today. It is
therefore foolish not to seek the help of a doctor in these

instances. Another interesting variation in pattern is found among women who dislike intercourse. They are apt to develop prolonged menstrual bleeding. If their husbands are away for a month or two the duration of menstruation may be restored to its normal length during their absence, only to become prolonged again on their return.

We have already mentioned travel abroad as a potent influence; similar environmental changes occur when young people enter college, take up nursing or enroll in the women's services, and may be followed by complete absence of menstruation for a few months while the body adjusts to the new environment. It is important to remember that the other systems in the body also take time to adjust to environmental change. Difficulty in getting to sleep, irregularity of bowel habit, alteration in appetite and weight are common complaints even on vacation.

Other stresses which alter the menstrual clock are stimulated by an adrenal hormone response. This can occur when the body's defense mechanism has been fighting an acute infection like pneumonia. At such times the corticosteroids produced by the adrenals stimulate the clock and alter the rhythm. The precise alteration experienced is again individual and variable; some respond to acute infection by temporarily missing menstruation, others by shortening the cycle and yet others by heavy or prolonged loss.

With all these influences producing so many variations in the menstrual pattern, it is not surprising that down through the centuries from the earliest times have come a multiplicity of theories that have produced a fascinating collection of folklore.

# 5

# Myths, Menstruation and Religion

Primitive man found menstruation hard to understand. The fact that month after month women lost blood and yet neither illness nor death followed mystified him, and for this reason many supernatural qualities were ascribed to it, both good and bad. Even today many men are amazed that women can accept the regular loss of blood so cheerfully, when they themselves are terrified each time they have a nosebleed or cut finger.

When primitive tribes lived in isolation there might be only one menstruating woman present at any one time. It was therefore natural to endow her with supernatural powers, normally ascribed only to their gods. These powers included her ability to stop hailstorms, whirlwinds or lightning if she went out into the open unclothed. The Italians believed that by encircling an olive grove infested with caterpillars, a menstruating woman could cause the insects to die. But the gathering together of large populations soon caused such myths to disappear.

The Hebrew described the menstruating woman by the word "tawny" or "taboo," a word which was also used to describe priests, "a holy taboo."

Menstrual blood was also thought to be endowed with valuable protective properties, being able to extinguish fires, temper metals and fashion swords as well as protecting men against wounds in battle. A thread soaked in menstrual blood was considered a valuable treatment for epilepsy or headache. It is, of course, recognized that a woman suffering from premenstrual epilepsy or headache will find relief as soon as she starts to menstruate. Is there a link here with the frequency with which premenstrual epilepsy, migraine and other premenstrual symptoms disappear when (as is mentioned in Chapter 9) the full flow of menstrual blood is established?

The presence of a menstruating woman was believed to cause much harm. She was supposed to be able to sour wines, blight crops, rust iron and bronze, turn copper green. She could also cause cattle to abort, seeds to dry up, fruit on trees to die, bright mirrors to become dulled, the edge to be taken off sharpened metals, the gleam of ivory to be dulled, a hive of bees to perish, needles and strings of harps and violins to break, clocks to stop and boiling linen to turn black. These ideas of the many and varied harmful effects of menstruating women make it easier to understand the practice of some Indian women going into purdah during these times.

The menstruating woman was thought also to bring about even worse disasters in certain circumstances. For instance should a menstruating woman walk between two men, then one of them would be certain to die. This placed upon menstruating women certain responsibilities, such as taking care not to touch fish or game when walking through streams or fields, lest the animal should later be caught by the hunters who then might die. In the forests she would call out to warn men of her presence so that they might avoid her, for should the man see a menstruating woman he would turn grey and lose his strength. In some communities women were isolated from the sight of men during these important days in specially reserved rooms, they were fed from vessels which needed to be destroyed after use, or else subjected to ritual purification.

During the Middle Ages it was believed that menstruation demonstrated the essential sinfulness and inferiority of women, and therefore menstruating women were forbidden to attend church or take communion, a custom which is still continued in some parts of the world today. Women of the Russian Orthodox Church are not permitted to kiss the cross or take communion during menstruation.

The Indians of Bolivia believed that menstruation resulted from the bite of a serpent or snake, and therefore following a woman's first menstruation there was a ritualistic beating of all household objects to kill the snake which had harmed the girl.

In Italy scanty menstruation was thought to be particularly harmful, and the accumulating blood was thought to cause madness and tuberculosis.

Intercourse during menstruation has long been thought to be harmful, as it was believed that the impurities of the body in the menstrual blood would foul the semen and so produce deformed or sickly babies with epilepsy or insanity. For this reason Orthodox Jewish women were instructed to make themselves plain and unattractive during menstruation to avoid exciting their husbands sexually. Following menstruation the woman was required to undergo a ritualistic cleansing. Full instructions are to be found in Leviticus, Chapter 15. A bath was taken in which the woman immersed herself three times in a "body of living water."

In different countries there are many local customs, each concerned chiefly with the local industry and fears of its failure. In Indonesia menstruating women may not enter tobacco fields or work in rice paddies. In Saigon they are not employed in opium factories, lest the opium turn bitter. In France and Germany they were excluded from the wineries and breweries lest they turn the wine or beer sour. In France it was feared that the presence of menstruating women during the boiling process in sugar refineries might turn the sugar black. Parsees in India may not look at a fire lest their glance extinguish it. In Syria it is feared that pickling done by menstruating women will cause the food to putrefy. Many countries in Southern Europe prohibited menstruating women from kneading or baking bread or cakes for this would prevent them from rising. Even the mere breath of a menstruating woman is thought, in the South of France, sufficient to prevent the mayonnaise from thickening. In South Africa menstruating women may not come in contact with cattle for fear they will turn the milk sour. In England, too, in the last century it was believed that if menstruating women salted meat it would not keep.

Many women, having made a sponge cake which failed to rise, a meringue which would not whip or jam which would not jell, will now look at their menstrual charts and appreciate the possible grain of truth in these menstrual myths. It is a time when women are more impatient, slap-dash and haphazard, and their work suffers. This aspect is dealt with more fully in later chapters.

These dangers are considered to be markedly increased with the first menstruations at puberty and unusual precautions were taken to isolate girls at these times. Sir James Frazer, in *The Golden Bough,* gives a fascinating account of the efforts made to prevent such girls touching the earth or seeing the sun. These vary from seclusion on a layer of banana leaves in a darkened house, practiced by a tribe near Lake Nyassa; in a suspended cage in New Ireland; on a house raised on piles in Borneo; to living in a specially constructed gallery of the house in Vancouver Island or enveloped in a hammock and slung from the roof in South America.

The period of seclusion at puberty varied, but within each tribe the rules appear to have been quite rigid. The Hindu girl's seclusion lasted only four days; in the Caroline Islands girls were isolated for several days, and in North Queensland the period of banishment lasted from four to six weeks. The Indians of Vancouver Island extended the spell to eight months. The longest seclusion was among tribes in New Ireland where it lasted four or five years and in Borneo where it continued for a full seven years. During the seclusion special foods, often fish and meat, were forbidden and eating was from special utensils which must later be destroyed; and the food was served by named individuals such as a slave, an old lady, a maternal aunt or one unable to bear a child. The end of seclusion was marked by celebrations during which the young girl might be immersed in water, beaten with twigs, decorated and covered with flowers or even exposed to the bites of certain large ants. These practices were performed to make her clean, so that she might mix once more with other people.

Even today there are some less progressive parents who forbid their daughters to take a bath or wash their hair during menstruation. To appreciate the origin of these ideas it is perhaps as well to recall the difficulty of both these tasks in the days before bathrooms, hot water and hair dryers existed. The cold water was a chilling experience and fears of catching a "death of a cold" naturally accompanied these tasks—more so when the women were losing warm menstrual blood. Perhaps the old wives of these tales recognized woman's lowered resistance to infections, only recently confirmed by medical research (see page 128). But of course there is no risk entailed in carrying out the normal procedures of hygiene, especially under modern conditions.

There are still far too many primitive theories about

menstruation locked up in people's minds. These will only be dispelled by the careful record-keeping and keen clinical observation of doctors as they study the women who come to their offices.

# 6

# The Doctor's Examination

When a doctor has finished the medical examination of a patient he will enter his finding on the patient's medical record card. Often he will use the letters "n.a.d." indicating "no abnormality detected," and meaning that on examination the patient appeared normal. Sometimes patients are confused by being told that all is normal, when they continue to have period pains. It should be appreciated that, although the doctor may not have been able to detect anything abnormal, it does not necessarily mean that everything is working exactly as it should. This book deals with those reasons for pain and symptoms for which no abnormality has been detected on full medical and gynecological examination.

Some people are shy and others are fearful of undergoing a full medical examination. Perhaps this is because they do not appreciate how important it is for the doctor to have a clear picture of the patient's physical condition, besides a full history of any past minor, as well as major, illnesses. The first part of the doctor's examination will no doubt be spent in carefully taking a history, or asking numerous questions about the patient's present health, past illnesses, the health of the husband and the family, about previous pregnancies, the usual menstrual pattern, habits of eating, smoking and drinking and also asking about the patient's life in general. Throughout this history-taking the doctor will be obtaining many useful pointers. He may even underline some of the facts that have emerged from the history to remind him to pay special attention to these in future. For instance, if there has been jaundice this will need special consideration in any future use of hormone therapy. Pulmonary tuberculosis in childhood may have left a focus of latent tuberculosis in the womb. Peritonitis in the distant past suggests the possibility of adhesions or chronic inflammation of the Fallopian tubes now. The doctor is interested in the family health, particularly in respect of high blood pressure, diabetes and other familial complaints. A severe hemorrhage following childbirth may result in subsequent hormonal upset, and if the pregnancy was complicated by toxemia then the blood pressure may still be unduly high. He is interested in whether the weight is stationary, increasing or decreasing. Loss of weight, while the appetite remains good, would suggest the need to eliminate the possibility of thyroid overactivity, diabetes or depression; while loss of weight and a poor appetite could suggest more generalized poisoning such as tuberculosis or cancer. A poor diet predisposes to anemia and nutritional diseases.

It has been known for a patient to complain that the doctor "wasted" a lot of time just talking and prying into her private life. A sincere and conscientious doctor will gain most valuable information from his introductory questions, so it is always in the patient's interest to cooperate and answer his questions fully.

The next stage of the examination will take place on the examining couch. At the initial glance the doctor will sum up the extent of the secondary sex characteristics and determine how this conforms with the typical feminine appearance. Figure 8 shows the signs of feminine development including the axillary and pubic hair and the

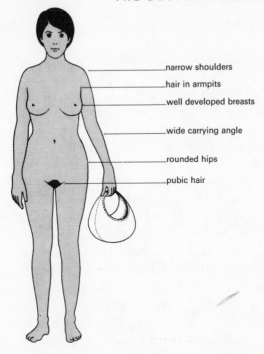

narrow shoulders

hair in armpits

well developed breasts

wide carrying angle

rounded hips

pubic hair

Figure 8. Feminine characteristics

breasts; any one of these features may be undeveloped, normal or overdeveloped. The male is characterized by a different hair distribution especially on the thighs, chest and abdomen. Men have broad shoulders and narrow hips, while the more a woman resembles the rounded figure of Renoir's women the more feminine she will look. When women hold their arms down and palms facing to the front they have a larger "carrying" angle at the elbows than have the men. It is known as the "carrying" angle because it enables the woman to carry pails, baskets, parcels, hanging clear from the side of the thigh and therefore more easily than is possible for a man. A rough assessment of the probable size of the pelvis and consequently the ease of labor in childbirth can be made from consideration of the roundness or flatness of the hips and pelvis.

The general examination will probably include looking at the membranes of the eyes to determine whether there is any hint of anemia; if there is, special blood tests will be arranged. The blood pressure will be taken, and again if this is raised some further blood and kidney tests may be advisable. The stethoscope will be used to eliminate possibilities of diseases of the heart or lungs. A clean tongue suggests a clean bill of health for the digestive system. Meanwhile the presence or absence of obesity, acne, varicose veins, old operation scars and skin lesions will be observed. Any hint of puffiness around the ankles will be carefully examined with pressure of the finger to see whether it leaves an indentation, suggesting the presence of edema or excess fluid in the tissues; simple fat leaves no indentation after pressure.

Normally the womb is too small to be felt on examination of the abdomen, for it is hidden behind the pubic bone. If the womb is enlarged because of pregnancy, fibroids or any other abnormality, then it can be felt rising up out of the pelvis and its size, shape and consistency will be carefully noted. Similarly the ovaries cannot be detected, except when they are enlarged because of ovarian cysts or growths. The liver, spleen and kidneys cannot be felt except when diseased, but the areas in which these enlarged organs might be present will be carefully palpated. This means that the hand will be gently laid on the area to feel for any abnormality. Normally there should be no tenderness on examination of the abdomen, but if any is found its exact position and extent will be noted and further tests will be needed.

To the uninitiated the idea of an internal examination may seem frightening. In actual fact it is a very simple and easy procedure completed in two or three minutes, and should never be accompanied by pain. The single girl would have the position, size and shape of her womb estimated by examination through her rectum, as her hymen will block entry to the vagina. Should a further examination be needed, particularly if examination of the ovaries is required, then she might be asked to go into a hospital overnight so that she can be fully examined under an anesthetic.

The married woman is easier to examine; since she has had sexual intercourse, the entry of the doctor's finger or instruments can be accomplished painlessly. The size, shape and position of the womb will be estimated, and the neck of the womb will be inspected directly. At the same time the doctor will probably take a cervical smear or cancer test of the neck of the womb, and possibly also a vaginal swab to test for the presence of any bacteria in the vagina. Healthy ovaries cannot be felt, but an attempt will be made to determine whether they are enlarged or abnormal in any other way.

In most cases where women are attending for menstrual symptoms, the examinations just mentioned will show no abnormality. Occasionally fibroids may be detected, there may be an ulcer or erosion at the neck of the womb, ovarian cysts may be found, or the presence of infected Fallopian tubes, or cancer of the womb, ovaries or vagina may be suspected. All these will require further investigations and are outside the scope of this book. Sometimes, especially in the case of an older woman with menstrual irregularity, although the above-mentioned examinations are all quite normal, the doctor may, for various reasons, consider it wise for her to be admitted to a hospital for a special examination under anesthesia during which scrapings are taken from the lining of the womb for microscopic examination to exclude any possibility of cancer lurking within the body of the womb.

In spite of all the possibilities that have been mentioned in this chapter, the greater majority of women will go through all these examinations without any abnormality being detected.

# 7

# Period Pain

The idea of painless menstruation has been described by one sufferer as a "figment of male imagination." Estimates of the frequency of suffering among women in whom the monthly pains are severe enough to interfere with normal working capacity and enjoyment of life, vary from five to eight in every ten women. One medical colleague excused the present neglect of sufferers of *dysmenorrhea,* or period pains, by saying that as they had "n.a.d." on their notes after full examination it was assumed that they must be suffering from a purely psychological complaint.

In this decade of synthetic hormone therapy the problem of period pain is easy enough to cope with. Biochemists are endeavoring to find a simple test to obtain an assessment of the precise amount of hormones circulating in the blood at any particular time of the menstrual cycle. This might enable them to make an exact determination of the degree and type of dysmenorrhea as well as the precise hormone required to alleviate the pain.

There are two very different and, in fact, opposite types of dysmenorrhea, known as *spasmodic* and *congestive.* "Spasmodic" gets its name from the spasms of pain and "congestive" from the belief that pain was caused by blood congestion, although it is now known to be due to water retention. It is vital to determine at the beginning the type of dysmenorrhea from which the patient is suffering, for the hormone treatment of the two types is quite different. If the wrong hormone is given it may well increase the pain. In fact dysmenorrhea can be induced in any woman by the administration of the wrong hormone. This invalidates any theory that dysmenorrhea is purely psychological.

Dysmenorrhea means pain with periods but tells us no more than this and is no guide to treatment. The type of pain and the precise time at which it actually occurs decide the type of dysmenorrhea (Figure 9).

*Spasmodic dysmenorrhea.* This has the onset of pain strictly on the first day, although it may continue for the next two or three days. The pain is most severe on the first day, coming on within an hour of the first sign of menstrual flow. It is usually felt as spasms of acute colicky pains in the lower abdomen. Although the pain may become dull, every twenty minutes or so it may suddenly without warning become acute again for another few minutes. During the spasms the pain is eased by bending over or curling up in a ball. The most comfortable position is curled up in bed hugging a hot water bottle. The spasms of pain may be severe enough to cause vomiting, or fainting, and they resemble labor pains in type and position. As the pain is strictly limited to those parts of the body controlled by the uterine or ovarian nerves, it may be in the back, inner sides of the thighs and lower abdomen, but not in other distant parts of the body such as the breasts, head, hands or feet. There may be individual exceptions, but sufferers from spasmodic dysmenorrhea tend to be immature, shy, with pale nipples, small breasts and scanty pubic hair.

Spasmodic dysmenorrhea is commonest between the ages of fifteen and twenty-five years, but it is not definitely limited to those ages only. It is rare for the first few men-

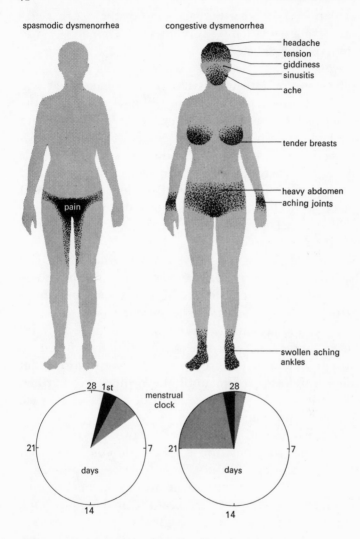

Figure 9. Time and site of symptoms

struations at puberty to be accompanied by spasmodic dysmenorrhea; the reason is thought to be that during the early years of menstruation, ovulation does not occur, and the onset of painful periods is due to the occurrence of ovulation. This is further borne out by the fact that suppression of ovulation by hormones will temporarily cure this type of dysmenorrhea.

*Congestive dysmenorrhea* is the opposite type, closely related to, or rather a variation of, premenstrual syndrome. In this type the woman will have warning of the onset of menstruation for several days, possibly even a week, during which she will experience increasing heaviness and a dull aching pain in the lower abdomen. This pain may be accompanied by nausea, lack of appetite and constipation. The premenstrual tension symptoms will make her feel exhausted, irritable and depressed. Headache, backache, and breast pains are a common accompaniment.

The sufferers of congestive dysmenorrhea often tend to have large breasts, dark brown nipples, ample pubic and axillary hair, rounded feminine hips and female bone structure. They also tend to be the women desiring large families and possessing marked maternal instincts. They may date the onset of dysmenorrhea from their first menstruations and may continue with the pains throughout their childbearing life until the menopause. Further, their dysmenorrhea will tend to be increased by each successive pregnancy.

When differentiating between the two types of dysmenorrhea the vital question is, "How do you know your period is coming?" If the sufferer looks vague, answering merely, "Oh I look at the calendar," or wonders why such a stupid question is being asked, she obviously does not get the warning symptoms diagnostic of congestive dysmenorrhea. When another woman is asked the same question, it may well be the husband or mother who answers, saying, "All the household knows when it's coming—she's so bad-tempered and irritable," or they may describe the warning symptoms of premenstrual tension. This woman is suffering from congestive dysmenorrhea.

There tends to be a family likeness in the type of dysmenorrhea suffered by mother and daughter; they both may be of the spasmodic type or both congestive. This is perhaps why unsympathetic advisers are apt to blame the mother for unwittingly having communicated her anxieties and pain about menstruation to her daughter.

Another group of menstrual problems are combined under the omnibus title of *premenstrual syndrome*. The word "syndrome" means a group of symptoms occurring together. Premenstrual syndrome covers those symptoms which recur with each menstruation. These symptoms may include pain or congestive dysmenorrhea but often pain is absent. The more important symptoms are premenstrual tension (which covers the triad of depression, irritability and lethargy), headaches, breast pains, joint pains, backache, acne, epilepsy, hay fever and asthma.

In a questionnaire study of a random sample of the general population of English women, Drs. N. Kessel and A. Coppen found that spasmodic dysmenorrhea was not associated with a particular psychological type, nor was the sufferer more neurotic than other women. They did find that those with premenstrual tension tended to be more neurotic. However, in their study they assessed how neurotic a woman was by the number of different symptoms she complained of and later chapters explain that an important characteristic of premenstrual syndrome and of water retention is that it causes numerous and varying symptoms. Therefore, when a woman with premenstrual syndrome is assessed on such a questionnaire, she will be considered "neurotic." Fortunately this is a classification which disappears with the successful treatment of the symptoms of premenstrual syndrome.

The cause of the two different types of dysmenorrhea is explained by the relatively different levels of circulating ovarian hormones, estrogen and progesterone. Figure 10 shows arbitrary levels of estrogen and progesterone dia-

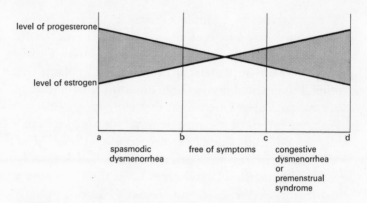

Figure 10. Arbitrary levels of progesterone and estrogen

grammatically. Patients with their progesterone levels markedly raised above the estrogen level, as in the shaded area AB, are liable to suffer from spasmodic dysmenorrhea, and those whose estrogen levels are markedly raised above the progesterone levels as in the shaded area CD, are liable to suffer from congestive dysmenorrhea or premenstrual syndrome. Patients with only a slight variation between the levels of the two ovarian hormones, in the area BC, are likely to be free from these menstrual disorders.

Consideration of this diagram makes it clear that the two types of menstrual pains are at the opposite poles of normality. The degrees of severity pass from severe spasmodic dysmenorrhea, through mild spasmodic dysmenorrhea to normality, and on to mild congestive dysmenorrhea or premenstrual syndrome to severe congestive dysmenorrhea or premenstrual syndrome. It becomes obvious now why it is vital to differentiate between the two types, and why they require the opposite hormone therapy. Spasmodic dysmenorrhea requires estrogen therapy and congestive dysmenorrhea requires progesterone therapy.

The diagram also explains why administration of excessive quantities of either estrogen or progesterone to a woman who is normally symptom free, with hormone levels in the shaded area BC, may alter these levels to bring her within the shaded area CD, giving premenstrual syndrome or into the area AB, giving her spasmodic dysmenorrhea. When estrogen is taken in the form of the Pill by a woman whose hormone levels are in the shaded area CD it can produce unwanted side effects or even prove dangerous.

# 8

# Treatment of Spasmodic Dysmenorrhea

As mentioned previously the treatment of the two types of dysmenorrhea is quite different. Because the treatment of congestive dysmenorrhea is the same as for premenstrual syndrome, consideration of this type of dysmenorrhea has been postponed to Chapter 11.

Figure 10 on page 44 suggests that the cause of spasmodic dysmenorrhea is a relative excess of progesterone compared with estrogens. This may be an over-simplification which will possibly need modifying when more is known about the interaction of the numerous corticosteroids. Nevertheless, it is true that the relief of spasmodic dysmenorrhea can be accomplished by the administration of estrogens.

Fortunately the estrogen hormones can be given by mouth and are easily used by the body. The dose varies for each individual and may have to be found by trial and error. Once an ideal dose for one patient is found, this dose may need to be given for several months; then the dose can gradually be reduced over the next few months and finally stopped.

Each doctor has his favorite brand of estrogen which he finds works best in his hands. The actual type of estrogen used is not so important as the finding of each patient's ideal dose. The amount of estrogen required to relieve spasmodic dysmenorrhea is usually well below that contained in the contraceptive pills, and indeed the dose rarely exceeds 50 micrograms, which is the maximum permitted in the Pill in Britain. What is important is that the estrogen is given to correct a hormone imbalance in an estrogen-deficient woman, which is quite different from the taking of estrogen in a Pill by a woman who already has an estrogen sufficiency or even surplus.

When analyzing the replies sent in to the *Which?* inquiry about period pains, several patients wrote that they received relief of pains when on hormones, but the next month the pains were just as bad. This is true. Unfortunately it is necessary to continue the estrogen therapy for several months and the patient should appreciate this at the beginning of treatment.

The author's view is that estrogen therapy serves to increase the size and general muscular development of the womb. It would obviously take several months to show any significant growth, and this would explain why it is possible after a few months to lower the dose of estrogen and still get the same beneficial effect. Ultimately, when the womb is of sufficient size, the estrogen therapy can be discontinued and further treatment becomes unnecessary.

The added advantage which estrogen therapy brings to patients with spasmodic dysmenorrhea is the automatic regulation of the menstrual cycle to about every twenty-eight days and the certainty of moderate bleeding. Those whose cycles are normally unduly short or excessively long, and those who feel they are losing too heavily or only an insignificant amount are delighted to have these other inconveniences relieved at the same time as bringing relief of their monthly incapacity and pain.

Estrogen therapy does prevent ovulation, so it cannot be used in the treatment pattern, already mentioned, for those eager to conceive. Such patients benefit from estrogen given on days 16–27, that is, after ovulation has occurred. The subsequent relief is not so complete as with the more prolonged course of estrogen, and usually a larger dose of estrogen is necessary.

Contraceptive pills contain estrogens and progestogens and are used in a course of treatment on days 5–25. They are excellent in curing spasmodic dysmenorrhea and can be used in preference to estrogen alone in those patients anxious not to conceive.

During treatment patients should record on their menstrual charts the presence or absence of pain each month as this serves as a most useful guide for the control and adequacy of treatment.

In the majority of women complaining of menstrual pain it is easy enough by careful questioning to distinguish between the two types of dysmenorrhea, spasmodic or congestive. However, occasionally diagnosis is not clearcut, especially for patients whose mother tongue is not English and from whom a clear history cannot be obtained. It is possible to give such patients a menstrual chart to use for a couple of months while they are receiving other pain-relieving tablets, or one can give a therapeutic trial. This means giving the patient a trial with estrogen in the usual dosage on days 5–25, and if the subsequent menstruation is pain-free one can assume that the dysmenorrhea is of the spasmodic type. On the other hand if the patient has congestive dysmenorrhea estrogen will increase the subsequent dysmenorrhea. Fortunately there is a natural safety valve here, for when estrogen is used on patients with congestive dysmenorrhea (who already have high estrogen levels) the added estrogen causes nausea after only two or three days. Such patients are therefore instructed to take the tablets from day 5 of the cycle, but to stop immediately if there is any sign of nausea or other side effects. Those patients who develop nausea with estrogen would then be treated for congestive dysmenorrhea as described in Chapter 11.

Occasionally patients with spasmodic dysmenorrhea are advised to have a small operation called D & C. This means dilatation of the neck of the womb under an anesthetic. It gives relief to spasmodic dysmenorrhea, but never to congestive dysmenorrhea. Unfortunately in this operation the mouth of the womb is very occasionally over-stretched, and in a few patients this may cause difficulty in maintaining any subsequent pregnancies. Sometimes a D & C is needed to assist diagnosis and eliminate the possibility of polyps or other growths in the womb.

Undoubtedly patients suffer more pain when in poor than when in good health, therefore the general advice of having plenty of sleep, good food and ample exercise may make a difference to the degree of incapacity and pain, but it is unlikely to change dysmenorrhea to a complete absence of pain.

Many are advised to lead more active lives, but the *Which?* survey showed that only a third of the sufferers of spasmodic dysmenorrhea had sedentary occupations. When they kept menstrual charts during their vacations women were asked specifically to record if the dysmenorrhea increased or decreased in severity. Many went on vacations which were more active than their usual life, e.g. canoeing or hiking, while others chose more relaxing vacations by the Mediterranean, but the common pattern was to find that the dysmenorrhea was unaffected by vacations, the pain occurring for as long as usual and at the same time in relation to menstruation. One can't help feeling sympathy for the school games captain and winner of the *victrix ludorum* who said, "Please don't tell me the pain will go if I take more exercise."

On the other hand there is a scheme of relaxation and exercises which has been devised by Mrs. Erna Wright.

This is based on the same principle as painless child-birth, namely that full knowledge of the reproductive processes plus exercises for the vital muscles and the ability to relax will be helpful in removing some period pains. The scheme of exercises is simple enough and some may prefer to try them for a month or two before commencing hormone therapy.

It will be noticed that all the methods of treatment given so far deal with prevention of an attack well in advance. During an actual attack of pain the sufferer gets most relief from a warm bath, followed by a rest in bed with a hot water bottle. An aspirin, paracetamol or codeine may relieve the spasms, while on the odd occasion the relief obtained from a sip of brandy or rum is astonishing. Food is not essential, and the sufferer is probably better left to sleep it off quietly, rather than having food pressed on her, which may induce nausea or vomiting.

The problems of congestive dysmenorrhea and the premenstrual syndrome will be considered in the next chapter.

# 9

# Premenstrual Syndrome

Our understanding of premenstrual syndrome is still in its early years. It was as recently as 1953 that Dr. Raymond Greene and the author wrote the first article on the subject in the British medical press. This first article contained the case histories of eighty-seven women sufferers with an analysis of their characteristics. At that time the joint authors had little idea that what was being described covered the habits and changeable personalities of at least half the female population, nor that its influence was worldwide.

Premenstrual syndrome covers a wide variety of cyclical symptoms which regularly recur at the same phase of the menstrual cycle. The commonest time for their recurrence is during the few days before menstruation, hence the title, but they may continue until the full menstrual bleeding has begun. Occasionally they occur during ovulation. The onset of full menstruation usually brings swift and dramatic relief, but as there may be only a slight menstrual loss for a day or two before the full bleeding begins, it is not uncommon for the symptoms to persist through the first day or two of each cycle.

The symptoms which can be found in premenstrual syndrome are extraordinarily varied and there are few tissues in the body which may not on occasions be affected by menstrual variations and premenstrual aggravations. The diagnosis of premenstrual syndrome is dependent on the cyclical reappearance of the symptoms at the same phase of each menstrual cycle. This is where the menstrual charts are invaluable. The patient is asked to record her symptoms by using such signs as "H" for headache, "B" for backache and "X" for pains, acne, asthma, epilepsy or quarrels. (Few women like to record accurately for all the world to see the dates of their quarrels, but the universal "X" which can mean several different symptoms is easily understood by the doctor.) Capital letters can be used for severe attacks of headaches and backaches and the small letters for milder attacks. Clumping together of symptoms about the time of menstruation is instantly recognized on a menstrual chart (Figure 11).

An essential feature of the diagnosis of premenstrual syndrome is the presence of a few days, always the same days in each menstrual cycle, when the woman is completely free from symptoms. Sometimes attacks occur at ovulation but premenstrual symptoms always also follow. These attacks may merge into one prolonged attack from ovulation to menstruation with a symptom-free phase during the postmenstruum. One unfortunate Irish woman complained, "I only feel well when I'm poorly."

Occasionally women will speak mistakenly of "postmenstrual tension." Examination of their menstrual charts will show either that the symptoms have no relationship to menstruation but are related to external stress; or that the symptoms are an extension of a premenstrual or menstrual attack which has continued into the first day of the postmenstruum. Sometimes because the attack occurs at ovulation, which is nearer the last day of menstruation than to the beginning of the next menstruation, it is erroneously regarded as postmenstrual.

When other premenstrual symptoms are present, premenstrual tension will be the invariable accompaniment.

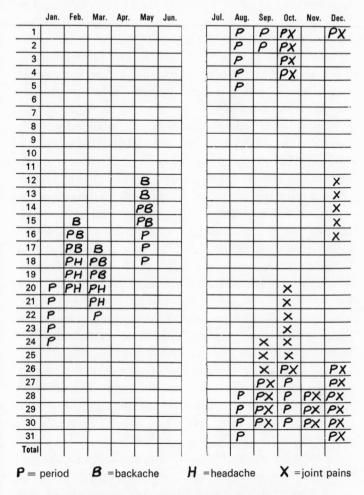

P = period  B = backache  H = headache  X = joint pains

Figure 11. Menstrual charts showing premenstrual syndrome

Sometimes a patient will attend with an apparently small recurrent premenstrual problem, like a sty or shingles on the lip, and then burst into tears when describing how this one small spot is getting her down, losing her friends and taking away all her energy. In reality she has premenstrual tension, with its triad of irritability, depression and lethargy, in addition to the one blemish on the skin. Treatment of the premenstrual syndrome will relieve all her symptoms.

*Premenstrual tension* was aptly described by Dr. H. E. Billig in 1953 as "crabby" (irritability), "the world looks like a sour apple" (depression) and "a fall in energy" (lethargy).

*Irritability* is usually irrational, accompanied by little insight. The sufferer becomes agitated, impatient, jittery, explosive, intolerant, spiteful, bad-tempered or irrationally aggressive. She even wakes up in the morning feeling "at war with the world" and dreads the inevitable problems her day will produce. Her fiery outburst of irritability may bring her on the wrong side of the law, may cause a break-up of her marriage, may mean the end of her present job, or it may mean the loss of her friends. Then suddenly her irritability ends. She is once more her usual sweet-tempered and placid self, or she may be filled with guilt and remorse at the problems her actions have caused. One woman said, "I wish others would realize it wasn't the true me who caused all this."

In France it is recognized that premenstrual irritability may be so acute and irrational that for legal purposes it is regarded as a form of temporary insanity. In its mildest form the irritability may appear no more than "feminine contrariness."

*Depression* is manifested by weeping and a pessimistic outlook, often relieved by congenial company. It can be quite severe while it lasts, but the total duration is rarely more than a few days. Friends and workmates close to the woman may realize that this is not an opportune time to make plans or ask favors.

*Lethargy*, tiredness or exhaustion lasts only a few days. This is the type of symptom which brings a patient to the office for a medicine. The tiredness is both mental and physical. The widespread effect on schoolgirls' weekly work and examination performance will be referred to later, but workers on piecework are usually only too well aware of their temporary poor performance at routine tasks usually accomplished with ease. The physical tiredness may be overpowering, the housewife may return to her bed after her husband has left for work. One patient would lie on the park bench on her way to work in the mornings and sleep there. A sixteen-year-old girl at boarding school was referred for treatment after the Matron had found her sleeping at her desk while other girls were out playing. There is increased clumsiness and loss of manual dexterity, so that breakages increase markedly during the premenstruum.

Characteristically, patients with premenstrual syndrome have more than one symptom. Apart from tension, sufferers from premenstrual migraine may also complain of premenstrual bloatedness of the abdomen, breast tenderness and spells of giddiness. This presence of multiple symptoms leads to patients being wrongly classed "neurotic," as formerly were many sufferers from other endocrine disorders like diabetes, myxedema or Addison's disease, before biochemical investigations led to a positive diagnosis.

Among the commonest symptoms are headache (either the acute migraine attack or milder prolonged attacks), asthma, hay fever or allergic rhinitis, giddiness, fainting, epilepsy, joint and muscle pains, backache, skin lesions and inflammation of the eyes. The characteristic feature of these symptoms is the time relationship to menstruation. These symptoms of premenstrual syndrome cover every medical specialty and it is only the family doctor who sees the full spectrum of possibilities and combinations.

When the symptoms are centered on the lower abdomen there will be heavy, dragging premenstrual pain, which eases only with menstrual bleeding. This is congestive dysmenorrhea, so often accompanied by other symptoms of headache, breast pains, and the tension symptoms of irritability, depression and lethargy. But many sufferers from premenstrual syndrome have completely pain-free menstruations. These are the women who find it difficult to realize that their periodic attacks of migraine, epilepsy, asthma or depression should be associated with a menstruation in which there is no discomfort. These are also the women who require a menstrual chart for diagnosis, to convince them that their other recurrent and chronic symptoms are related to menstruation and can therefore be successfully treated.

During the premenstruum the patient may show edema or puffiness of the ankles, abdomen, fingers or face. Some complain that their dentures do not fit securely during the premenstruum, others find that while they can normally wear tight-fitting skirts they need a looser garment before menstruation. Some wear a specially loose-fitting pair of shoes, and yet others need two sizes of bra, one reserved for the premenstruum.

Food fads are common during the premenstruum, and are often similar to those experienced by the same woman during pregnancy. Often she desires crunchy foods, like cornflakes, raw cabbage, sprouts, or even charcoal, while another changes her normal preference for tea to a desire for strong black coffee.

Spontaneous bruising is frequent during the premenstruum because of the bursting of minute capillaries. These bruises appear even though there has been no injury. They are painless, usually all the same size and shape and circular in appearance. They are common on the thighs and upper arms. They become a possible danger at times of marital disharmony when the husband is wrongly accused of having hurt his wife and caused bruises, which are there for all to see.

Day-to-day observations of patients suffering from

severe premenstrual syndrome may show a slight but consistent rise in blood pressure during the premenstruum or menstruation. The rise may be about 20 to 30 mm. Hg (not high enough to bring an individual with normal blood pressure into the high blood pressure category). Similarly there may be a temporary gain of weight of about three to seven pounds. There was a report by Dr. W. A. Thomas in 1933 of a woman who gained twelve to fourteen pounds with each menstrual cycle, but this has been surpassed by a patient of Drs. E. and E. K. Novak, reported in 1952, who regularly gained fifteen pounds in weight during the premenstruum.

Regular observations of women suffering from glaucoma at the Institute of Ophthalmology, London, have shown that there is a premenstrual rise in intra-ocular pressure and also a simultaneous rise in blood pressure and weight (Figure 12). Each patient has her own individual timing of the rise. Some show the rise in the premenstruum followed by a drop during menstruation before returning to the intermenstrual level. Other women show a premenstrual drop followed by a marked menstrual rise before a return to normality. Apart from the eye symptoms the other symptoms like bloatedness, giddiness and tension occur at times when the blood pressure and body weight are highest. These individual patterns of premenstrual rises and menstrual drops in one, and premenstrual drops followed by menstrual rises in another woman, mean that when an average of several patients' weights, blood pressures, and intra-ocular pressure are taken the individual pattern is ironed out and the general pattern of menstrual influence becomes obscured.

In the same way, though the word *paramenstruum* is used to cover both the four days of the premenstruum and the first four days of menstruation, in practice no one person is susceptible throughout the whole eight days. Some

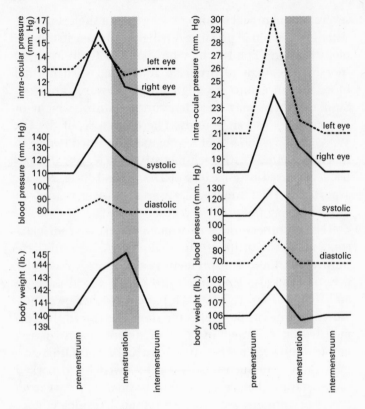

Figure 12. Influence of menstruation on glaucoma patients

find their tension greatest during the premenstruum, others during menstruation and yet others during the last two days of the premenstruum and the first two days of menstruation. But each woman soon enough recognizes the days on which she is likely to encounter most difficulties.

One marked characteristic of premenstrual syndrome is its similarity to toxemia of pregnancy. Both have the same signs of raised blood pressure, weight gain and edema, the one towards the end of the menstrual cycle, the other towards the end of pregnancy. In their severest form both can end in fits, either epileptic or eclamptic. Four out of five of those patients who have previously suffered from toxemia of pregnancy later develop premenstrual syndrome. Patients who have suffered from both premenstrual syndrome and toxemia of pregnancy tend to develop the same type of symptoms during the premenstruum as during later pregnancy. Thus one individual may develop headaches, backache and irritability, and another individual develop giddiness, vomiting and depression in both the premenstruum and during the pregnancy, becoming far worse towards the end of pregnancy. Further mention of toxemia is made in Chapter 17.

The severity of symptoms month by month may vary with stress. When a woman has had a particularly difficult month with domestic crises, legal problems or quarreling neighbors it is likely that her premenstrual symptoms will be increased. On the other hand a good win at the lottery may temporarily alleviate the symptoms for a sufferer of premenstrual syndrome.

# 10

# The Cause of Premenstrual Syndrome

Our knowledge of premenstrual syndrome has been gained only during the past fifteen years and it has been obtained from clinical observation, for unfortunately sex hormone and corticosteroid level estimations are still in their infancy. The following is a useful working hypothesis of the cause of premenstrual syndrome, and one must await further biochemical advance before it can be proved correct or becomes superseded by another theory.

Many, but not all, of the symptoms of premenstrual syndrome are characterized by water retention, an accumulation of excess cellular fluid. This would appear to be confirmed by the weight gain and decrease in volume of urine passed during the premenstruum when the symptoms are at their height, and the sudden weight loss and passing of large quantities of urine as the symptoms are relieved with menstruation.

The actual severity of the symptoms is not related to the total volume of water retained, judged by the weight gain, but rather by the position of the swollen cells. Thus a marked rise in pressure within the eye can result from a minute increase in the quantity of the natural fluid within the eye, an amount that would not be detected by weighing the whole patient. Whereas when the water is concentrated in the fat of the abdominal wall a large weight gain may occur with little discomfort.

Excessive quantities of water can be retained in any of the cells of the body. Wherever this occurs it can cause characteristic symptoms, such as tenderness when in the breasts, pain and headache in the sinuses, pain and glaucoma in the eyeballs, pain and edema in the ankles.

A common characteristic of women with premenstrual syndrome is that although they may be healthy, energetic and active women, they have great difficulty in standing still for long. This inability to stand for long periods is related to water retention and a tendency for the water (and blood) to accumulate in the feet, causing temporary cerebral anemia. It is immediately rectified by sitting or lying down and it does not occur when walking as the movement of the muscles inhibits the accumulation of fluid. These are the schoolgirls who faint after standing too long at morning assembly, and the women who edge themselves to the side of the room to lean against the walls at cocktail parties and other assemblies.

The actual site at which the water retention occurs is determined by four factors:

1. Anatomical abnormalities, such as narrow entrances to the sinuses which are easily blocked by engorged cells.

2. Heredity, such as the family predisposition to migraine.

3. Injury. Following a broken arm or leg it is common to find cyclical swelling occurring at the site many months after it has healed.

4. Infection. An upper respiratory infection could produce premenstrual engorgement of the sinuses instead of water retention at the patient's usual site in the breasts or abdomen.

The extra water that has been retained by the body

during the premenstruum is lost, sometimes within a few hours, by the passage of excess urine. Sometimes this wakes the sufferer up from sleep at night and she knows that she will be feeling better the next day. Occasionally the copious urine which is passed after an attack may be confused with menstrual blood, and the patient is worried that she is losing large quantities of blood with her urine.

But water retention does not account for all the symptoms of premenstrual syndrome; other groups of symptoms are accounted for by different mechanisms. The psychological symptoms of tension, irritability, depression and lethargy appear to be due to sodium retention and potassium depletion. There is too much sodium within the cells and too much potassium in the fluid bathing the cells. Premenstrual hay fever, urticaria and asthma are allergic phenomena. The faintness, weakness and sweating occurring premenstrually may be due to a spontaneous drop in the level of the blood sugar, or hypoglycemia. Recurrent infective episodes of sties, boils or herpes appear to be due to a lowering of the body's powers of resistance to bacteria and viruses.

Now consider the known facts:

1. The adrenal glands produce many corticosteroids, each with a different function. Some are responsible for the water balance in the tissues of the body, others regulate the sodium and potassium in the cells, some prevent allergic reactions, others regulate the level of the blood sugar and some mobilize mechanisms responsible for protection of the body from bacterial and viral infections.

2. In the adrenals progesterone is formed from simpler chemical compounds. The progesterone is the precursor, from which, after more chemical reactions, the many and varied corticosteroids are formed (Fig-

ure 13). Thus progesterone is present in the adrenals throughout the entire monthly cycle and it is the essential basis for all corticosteroids.

3. The ovary also produces progesterone, but only during the second half of the menstrual cycle, and its production ceases at menstruation.

4. When a patient with premenstrual syndrome is treated with progesterone from ovulation to menstruation, symptoms do not develop.

From these facts it is possible to produce a working hypothesis. It is suggested that if, during the premenstruum, the ovary produces insufficient progesterone for the requirements of the womb, some progesterone is taken from the other source, the adrenal glands, leaving them short for their production of corticosteroids. The balance of corticosteroids is temporarily upset and may result in water retention, imbalance of sodium and potassium, failure to control allergic reactions, alteration of the blood sugar level and lowered resistance to infection. All these mechanisms could account for the presence of the various premenstrual symptoms.

It would also account for the monthly recurrence of premenstrual syndrome in those whose womb or ovaries have been removed.

# 11

# Treatment of
# Premenstrual Syndrome

The correction of premenstrual syndrome is the correction of the water, sodium and salt potassium imbalance. This can be achieved by the administration of progesterone.

Progesterone, unfortunately unlike estrogen, cannot be administered by mouth. It is insoluable in water, so is dissolved in oil, and this type of injection must be given deep into the buttocks. However, a course of progesterone injections during the second half of the menstrual cycle works wonders, not only in removing the presenting symptoms, whether these are migraine, epilepsy, asthma or depression, but also in removing other hidden symptoms like premenstrual tension, restoring the woman's normal equanimity, charging her with fresh energy, an optimistic outlook and a calm personality. Many a husband has commented after the first course of injections that his wife is now more like the woman he knew at their marriage.

The injection will be needed daily or on alternate days and can be given by the district nurse, the nurse at work, the husband, or the patient herself. It is surprising that many a woman manages to inject herself after a short course of tuition. This has the added advantages of independence and the fact that she can give it to herself early in the day, which is usually the best time.

Sometimes when it has been proved that a course of injections is effective, a progesterone implant can be given. This is a very simple operation, performed under a local anesthetic, in which five to ten small pellets of pure progesterone are inserted into the fat of the abdominal wall or the thighs through a half-inch incision. An implant will last for between three and nine months. There may be painless and slight irregular menstrual bleeding during that time, but this may be considered a small price to pay for the removal of so many symptoms and relief from daily injections.

Progesterone has two functions in the body: first, that of building up the endometrial lining of the womb, and second, that of forming a base from which other adrenal corticosteroids are manufactured (Figure 13). Our biochemists are busy making synthetic progesterone-like preparations, called *progestogens*. The efficiency of any particular new progestogen is tested by its ability to build up the endometrium in rabbits and mice whose ovaries have been removed and who have already been given a course of estrogens. There are many effective progestogens, which can be taken by mouth and which have this property. They are most useful in those gynecological conditions in which the patient is not building up a good endometrium herself, and they are the basis of all contraceptive pills. But they do not have the dual ability possessed by the natural progesterone of being the basis for the formation of corticosteroids.

The action of progesterone is species specific. That means that it acts differently in different animal species. For instance, in humans progesterone causes an increased water and sodium excretion, which appears to be unique and is peculiar to humans. On the other hand, in dogs progesterone causes water and salt retention. It is be-

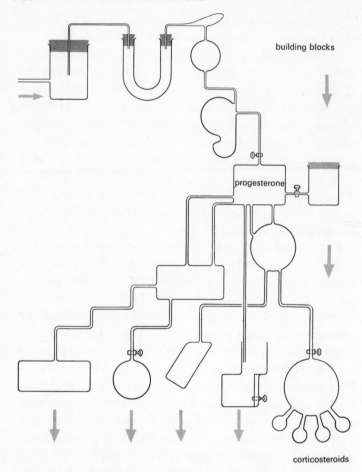

building blocks

progesterone

corticosteroids

Figure 13. Progesterone formation in the adrenals

cause of these variations among the species that a complete knowledge of the metabolism of progesterone in humans is not yet available. This is another problem the pharmaceutical industry has to contend with when testing new synthetic preparations of progestogens.

The chemical structure of estrogens, progesterone, testosterone and many of the adrenal corticosteroids is very similar. When a synthetic preparation like one of the progestogens is given, some women may find their bodies use it not only as a builder of the endometrium, but also as an estrogen, in which case it will cause nausea and increase the severity of the premenstrual syndrome. Alternatively they may find their bodies use it as an anabolic hormone, which increases tissue and causes them to put on weight. Yet other women may find that it is utilized in their bodies as a testosterone hormone and tends to produce male characteristics like hair growth. Occasionally the body may utilize the synthetic preparation as an aldosterone-antagonist like progesterone, in which case it will prove effective in preventing water retention. So it will be appreciated that the effect of each progestogen is personal to any given individual. While one progestogen may affect one person by increasing her premenstrual symptoms, another progestogen used on the same individual may remove her symptoms altogether. Therefore it is well worth trying on the patient several of the different oral progestogens, all with slightly different chemical formulas, to see if one of them will be effective in bringing relief of premenstrual syndrome.

Progestogens have a great advantage over progesterone injections in that they can be swallowed, but it may take some time before finding the ideal tablet for any one person. When a patient has severe symptoms and is at the end of her tether it is advisable to treat her first with a course of progesterone and to give her a month or two in which she can appreciate the joys of really good health, so that she knows what it means to be symptom free.

In addition to treatment with progesterone to correct the upset of water balance in the body, it is possible to remove the extra water retained in the body. Certain drugs, known as *diuretics,* have the ability to increase the output of urine, and if these are given they will remove the excess water that has been retained in the body. It is like baling water out of a leaking boat without sealing up the leak. It is the progesterone that stops the leak in the body. There are some highly effective diuretics on the market today; they can all be taken by mouth and can be used either alone or in addition to progesterone or progestogen therapy.

It has already been mentioned that the psychological symptoms of premenstrual tension are not due to the water retention but to an upset of the sodium and potassium balance. When diuretics are used to remove excess water in the body they tend also to remove potassium and to leave the excess sodium; therefore diuretics do not give relief to premenstrual depression, irritability or lethargy and may even increase the tension. In sufferers of premenstrual syndrome diuretics should only be given with the simultaneous administration of potassium, either alone or in one of the joint diuretic-potassium tablets.

In mild cases the patient can help herself by restricting her drinks to four cups of fluid per day during the last two weeks of each month and also restricting the salt in her diet. Strong coffee is a good diuretic, increasing the amount of urine passed, and many patients find themselves spontaneously drinking stronger and stronger coffee. While the premenstrual syndrome is being treated there is no need to stop the other more specific treatments for the individual symptoms. If a migraine sufferer gets relief from an ergometrine preparation during an attack there is no need to restrict it. An asthma sufferer may find that normally she is relieved by a bronchial dilator like ephedrine, or an epileptic by anti-convulsant drugs. These can all be continued at the beginning of progesterone or progestogen treatment, but when the woman is once fully stabilized on an efficient treatment she may disregard the ergometrine, ephedrine, or epanutin which were useful for her immediate symptoms.

Women's magazines give advice on period pains in their doctors' columns. Unfortunately this invariably seems to include suggestions that the sufferer should take excess fluids. "Drink two pints of water daily, preferably fresh cold water," or, "A glass of water when you wake will work wonders." It is difficult to know the origin of this old wives' tale but for women already waterlogged with congestive dysmenorrhea no benefit can result from this advice.

Already in this chapter we have discussed other well-intentioned but sometimes misguided treatments for premenstrual syndrome. It has been shown how the progestogens can be good or bad, and as these products are the basis of the Pill, designed to stop ovulation, it is perhaps time to discuss the subject of ovulation.

# 12

# Ovulation

At the midway point in the menstrual cycle the egg cell is released from one of the two ovaries and makes its way down the Fallopian tubes to the womb. This is normally a painless process and it is impossible for the average woman to know whether or when it is occurring. Very occasionally a patient comes for treatment because she has failed to become pregnant and in the course of the usual investigations into her infertility she may be astonished to learn that although she has been menstruating regularly no egg cell has been released from her ovaries during the months of observation.

The most convenient way of learning if ovulation is occurring in a particular woman is by asking her to take her temperature each morning for a month or two on waking and before getting out of bed. If examination of the temperature chart shows a rise of about one degree somewhere near mid-point between two menstruations this indicates that the woman is ovulating. The temperature may remain raised during the second half of the month, or it may revert to its former level. Both types are normal. Sometimes women are amazed at the day-to-day variation in their basal temperature and find the charts difficult to interpret themselves, in which case they should ask for the help of a doctor, especially if they are anxious to know precisely when they are ovulating.

Just occasionally women have slight bleeding or spotting of blood at ovulation. This is of no consequence, but unless it can be shown to be occurring regularly at midcycle it may be mistaken for irregular intermenstrual bleeding, which could be caused by something more serious like an ulcer on the neck of the womb, a polyp or a malignant growth (Figure 14). The bleeding is due to the sudden drop in the estrogen level at ovulation, and can be simply corrected by giving estrogen pills for three or four days before the expected time of bleeding. Treatment is needed only if the patient is really worried by its monthly recurrence; if she is content with the explanation that all is well, she will probably need no treatment.

Some adolescent girls get occasional abdominal pains in the left or right lower abdomen about two weeks after the start of menstruation. The pain is known as *Mittelschmerz* or "middle pain" and is due to ovulation. It can be easily recognized if marked on a menstrual chart (Figure 15) but is usually mistaken for appendicitis by the teenager. In fact, there is no vomiting or abdominal tenderness and the pain is never as severe as appendicitis. One girl went to the doctor with her bag packed, having convinced herself that she had appendicitis and would require immediate operation.

Occasionally in sufferers from premenstrual syndrome there may be a few short-lived symptoms at the time of ovulation, owing to the sudden change in ovarian hormone levels. There may be a migraine attack or asthmatic attack or just a day "off color." These are often the migraine sufferers who feel it unnecessary to keep a menstrual chart, as their migraine always occurs after menstruation, not before. In fact the menstrual record may confirm that it comes after menstruation, on about day 14. Fortunately migraine and other ovulatory symp-

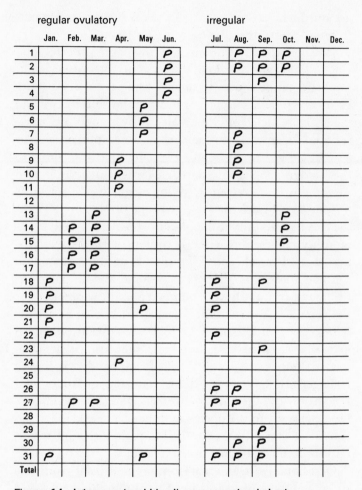

regular ovulatory                    irregular

| | Jan. | Feb. | Mar. | Apr. | May | Jun. | Jul. | Aug. | Sep. | Oct. | Nov. | Dec. |
|---|---|---|---|---|---|---|---|---|---|---|---|---|
| 1 | | | | | | P | | P | P | P | | |
| 2 | | | | | | P | | P | P | P | | |
| 3 | | | | | | P | | | P | | | |
| 4 | | | | | | P | | | | | | |
| 5 | | | | | P | | | | | | | |
| 6 | | | | | P | | | | | | | |
| 7 | | | | | P | | | P | | | | |
| 8 | | | | | | | | P | | | | |
| 9 | | | | P | | | | P | | | | |
| 10 | | | | P | | | | P | | | | |
| 11 | | | | P | | | | | | | | |
| 12 | | | | | | | | | | | | |
| 13 | | | P | | | | | | | P | | |
| 14 | | P | P | | | | | | | P | | |
| 15 | | P | P | | | | | | | P | | |
| 16 | | P | P | | | | | | | | | |
| 17 | | P | P | | | | | | | | | |
| 18 | P | | | | | | P | | P | | | |
| 19 | P | | | | | | P | | | | | |
| 20 | P | | | | P | | P | | | | | |
| 21 | P | | | | | | | | | | | |
| 22 | P | | | | | | P | | | | | |
| 23 | | | | | | | | | P | | | |
| 24 | | | | P | | | | | | | | |
| 25 | | | | | | | | | | | | |
| 26 | | | | | | | P | P | | | | |
| 27 | | P | P | | | | P | P | | | | |
| 28 | | | | | | | | | | | | |
| 29 | | | | | | | | | P | | | |
| 30 | | | | | | | | P | P | | | |
| 31 | P | | | | P | | P | P | P | | | |
| Total | | | | | | | | | | | | |

Figure 14. Intermenstrual bleeding on menstrual charts

toms respond admirably to progesterone therapy, but treatment must be started on about the seventh day of the cycle.

A medical social worker had been on contraceptive tablets for two years when she changed to a new brand to avoid side effects. At the fourteenth day of her cycle she mentioned to her husband, also in the medical field,

| | Jan. | Feb. | Mar. | Apr. | May | Jun. | Jul. | Aug. | Sep. | Oct. | Nov. | Dec. |
|---|---|---|---|---|---|---|---|---|---|---|---|---|
| 1 | | | | | | | | | | | | |
| 2 | | | | | | | | | | | | |
| 3 | | | | | | | | | | | | |
| 4 | | | | | | | P | | | | | |
| 5 | | | | | | | P | | | | | |
| 6 | | | | P | | | P | | | | | |
| 7 | | | | P | | P | | | | | | |
| 8 | | | | P | | P | | | | | | |
| 9 | | | | | P | P | | | | | | |
| 10 | | | | | P | P | | | | | | |
| 11 | | | | | P | | | | | | | |
| 12 | | | | | P | | | | | | | |
| 13 | | | | | P | | | | | | | |
| 14 | | | | | P | | | | | | | |
| 15 | | | | | | | | | | | | |
| 16 | | | | | | | | | | | | |
| 17 | | | | | | | X | | | | | |
| 18 | | | | | | | | | | | | |
| 19 | | | | X | | | | | | | | |
| 20 | | | | | X | | | | | | | |
| 21 | | | | | | | | | | | | |
| 22 | | | | | X | | | | | | | |
| 23 | | | | | | | | | | | | |
| 24 | | | | | | | | | | | | |
| 25 | | | | | | | | | | | | |
| 26 | | | | | | | | | | | | |
| 27 | | | | | | | | | | | | |
| 28 | | | | | | | | | | | | |
| 29 | | | | | | | | | | | | |
| 30 | | | | | | | | | | | | |
| 31 | | | | | | | | | | | | |
| Total | | | | | | | | | | | | |

Figure 15. Mittelschmerz shown on menstrual chart

that she felt sure she was ovulating because she had her usual mid-cycle symptoms. He did not believe this until in due course she became pregnant. The subsequent date of the birth of the baby strongly supported the view that conception probably occurred at the time the wife thought she was ovulating.

# 13

# The Pill

One of the most controversial subjects of this decade is the safety of the contraceptive pill. It is usually known as "The Pill" and always spoken of in the singular, although there would seem to be almost fifty-seven varieties of contraceptive tablet.

The Pill contains a combination of an estrogen and a progestogen in sufficient dosage to prevent ovulation. It is administered daily from the fifth day of the cycle for three weeks, there is then a break in taking the tablets for one week during which menstruation occurs, after which the Pill is restarted. There is little doubt that its effectiveness as a contraceptive measure is very near 100 per cent. Where contraception is desired, the Pill has many advantages over other methods like the male sheath, which requires last-minute preparations for natural expression of full love. It is infinitely preferable to the withdrawal technique, which leaves the woman frustrated and is rather like placing a delicious meal in front of a hungry person and, as she is about to eat, snatching it away from her. It avoids the careful calculation needed in the rhythm method. The Pill can be used by a woman who has had no children, whereas the other effective method of contraception, the intra-uterine device inserted into the womb, is suitable only for those who have had children.

Many things we habitually use have their risks, such as cars, stairs, boiling kettles and electricity; occasionally there may be an accident through using them and someone might be killed. All the enjoyable sports like car racing, skiing, football, swimming, have a risk, and just occasionally a fatality results. But, aware of the risk, we make our decision whether or not we participate. So too, whenever a doctor prescribes a drug, he must weigh up all the risks, for all drugs have a small risk. Aspirins, although millions are safely used daily, can very occasionally cause a stomach hemorrhage and result in death. Penicillin, the miracle and life-saving drug, can on very rare occasions cause sudden death from hypersensitivity. So too with the synthetic preparations contained in the Pill; just occasionally they can cause an unexpected death. If this happens, naturally the close relatives and friends will be strongly affected and will be anxious not to use the Pill or to see others use it. In the same way friends or relatives of a patient killed by aspirins or penicillin would naturally be wary if it were ever prescribed for them. It is always difficult to get a personal bereavement in true perspective.

Today, when so many anxieties are centered around the use of estrogen in the Pill it is important to remind the reader that during the past fifty years estrogen has been used regularly by doctors in the treatment of menstrual disorders. The dosage has always been carefully tailored for each patient and the problems of thrombosis have not occurred in these medically treated cases. This is very different from the mass administration of estrogen in the form of the Pill to healthy women, including those who already have high levels of natural estrogen (see pages 44–45). A parallel might be drawn with the other life-saving hormones, insulin and cortisone. These are valuable when given to a patient with known deficiency of the particular hormone, but would quickly prove lethal if given indiscriminately to everyone or made available from a slot machine.

There are certain indications which suggest that the doctor would be wise to avoid prescribing the Pill to certain women. These would be women with known liver or kidney disease or diabetes, those who have had jaundice (especially during a pregnancy), those with a history of thrombophlebitis, or with very large or inflamed veins, those who have needed treatment for cancer of the breast or womb. The Pill can be obtained only through a doctor; this is for general safety as he can then ask about the woman's present health and past illness before prescribing the Pill. Some patients not known to the doctor occasionally telephone asking the doctor to leave a prescription for the Pill for them to collect. They do not appreciate that the present requirement to obtain a prescription from a doctor, and not direct from the pharmacist, is for their own protection.

It has already been said that women with spasmodic dysmenorrhea respond readily to a course of estrogen therapy from the fifth day for three weeks. If they wish to avoid conception at the same time as receiving treatment for their period pains then the Pill is ideal for them. They will find that their period pains disappear and menstruation comes regularly every twenty-eight days with a small menstrual loss. Furthermore, if after a year or two they wish to conceive, they will probably find that on stopping the Pill their usual menstrual pattern returns but without period pains. These women are the ones who look better, brighter and more relaxed when taking the Pill.

On the other hand the story is quite different with those who suffer from congestive dysmenorrhea or from

premenstrual syndrome. These women require progesterone to relieve their symptoms. The Pill contains a progestogen, not progesterone. The progestogen may act on
any one individual as an estrogen, testosterone, anabolic
hormone or an aldosterone-antagonist (see pages 66–67).
If the particular progestogen in the Pill acts on an individual woman as an estrogen she will develop nausea and
an increase in premenstrual symptoms. If it acts as testosterone then it may cause hair growth of a masculine
distribution. If it acts as an anabolic hormone it results
in an increase in weight, always an unwanted symptom,
but unfortunately more likely to occur in those already
obese. On the other hand, when the progestogen acts as
an aldosterone-antagonist it can relieve premenstrual
water retention and restore general well-being to the
woman.

There have been reports of women who normally have
a slight premenstrual headache, but find that when they
start on the Pill they develop instead severe premenstrual
migraine. Others find that the Pill causes symptoms of
nausea, weight gain or giddiness. These are women whose
bodies mistake the progestogen in the Pill for some other
adrenal hormone. They would be well advised to change
their own particular brand of the Pill for some other
make. Each brand has its own different combination of
synthetic estrogen and progestogen, and if any diligent
woman searches long enough she should succeed in finding one brand which suits her requirements in every
respect. Recently in England the amount of estrogen
contained in the Pill has been limited to 50 micrograms.

A new pill containing progestogen only was marketed
but has since been withdrawn. Its action was not to in-
hibit ovulation, but to make the cervical secretion un-
acceptable to the male sperm. The ceaseless activity of
the pharmaceutical industry in its search for a safe oral
contraceptive may well lead to an oral preparation effec-

tive in relieving all symptoms of premenstrual syndrome.

Meanwhile many new and exciting trials are going on throughout the world to make family planning easier for the coming generation. Research workers are trying to find a "Morning-After Pill" which can be taken after intercourse, a "Once-a-Month Pill" to eliminate the need to take the other twenty tablets, a "Male Pill" to shift responsibility onto the man, or a three-monthly injection. Nevertheless there is still much to be learned about the ways in which the Pill works.

# 14

# Adjusting the Cycle

One of the unexpected bonuses received by all women on the Pill, or on a cyclical course of hormones, is
that they are given a cycle of precisely twenty-eight days
and that the loss is regulated so that it is not unduly heavy.
Some women on the Pill claim that the onset of menstruation is so regular they can even predict the exact hour
at which their menstruation will start. Doctors can alter
the menstrual clock. By the skilled use of hormones they
can make cycles as short as twenty days or as long as
desired, even up to a year or more without menstruation.

Hormone therapy has long been used to adjust the
cycle of those with very irregular and over-frequent menstruations and for those with unduly heavy or prolonged
menstruation. The hormones should be individually
tailored to suit the needs of each person, and will consist
either of estrogens or progestogens or a combination of
both. It may take a month or more while the ideal type
and dose is being found but, once found, the hormone
therapy can be used for months or years on end to regulate
menstruation to an acceptable pattern.

There are also medical occasions where it is desirable
to alter the menstrual pattern, and again hormone therapy can be used. Menstruation continues with para-
plegics, hemiplegics and other severely handicapped

women, yet, while chained to a hospital bed, their chances of pregnancy have vanished. In such women hormone treatment can usefully be given to prevent menstruation for the length of their incapacity. Dr. Anne Hamilton found that in such patients treatment was accompanied by an improvement in mental state, a feeling of well-being and a healing of bedsores. Women in plaster casts for fractured pelvis, spine or thigh bones would prefer to avoid the extra inconvenience of menstruation, even though their handicap is only temporary. They usually welcome the suggestion that their menstrual clock be halted until convalescence.

Women who find menstruation is due on their wedding night, during their annual vacation or when they are due to go into hospital for an operation, welcome an opportunity for either a shortening or lengthening of their menstrual cycle so that menstruation is avoided on these important occasions. A menstrual record is necessary to decide whether it would be wisest to bring menstruation forward or to delay its appearance.

Girls can be seriously handicapped at times of examinations if they have to take them during their paramenstruum (pages 114–17). Again the mere stress of examinations can be sufficient to change the usual menstrual pattern so that menstruation and examination coincide (pages 21–22). Candidates would be well-advised to give some thought to the timing of menstruation in relation to the coming examinations and if necessary to ask for medical advice on altering the timing of their menstrual clock.

It must be added that alteration of menstrual patterns is not permitted in respect of athletic events. This is because the male hormone, testosterone, has been known to be used. Testosterone has the effect not only of suppressing the feminine function of menstruation, but also of developing the masculine features of increased physical strength and endurance.

It is difficult to know where to draw the line when it comes to adjusting menstrual patterns. Most people would agree to assisting the handicapped. The woman astronaut obviously needs to be free of menstrual problems during her trip in space. Some may approve of the use of hormones for especially important events like weddings, and examination finals, and possibly too for the annual vacation for which they have been saving during the other fifty weeks of the year. How about the week-end yachting or sports car rally enthusiast? It is possible, easy, cheap and harmless to regulate her menstruation so that it always occurs midweek and leaves her free from Fridays to Sundays for her carefree enjoyment. Should this be considered a frivolous request, and, even if it is, should it be refused on that account?

Adult women looking back on the days of their youth must feel a little envious at the wonderful possibilities these new forms of treatment open up for the adolescents of the future.

# 15

# Adolescence

The onset of menstruation may be an exciting experience for a girl who longs for maturity and regards this feminine function as a sign of adulthood. It may be the reverse for an unprepared girl who one day to her surprise discovers she is bleeding and fears she is suffering from a frightening disease. In India it is the cause for a celebration, and the occasion is marked by the change from wearing short frocks to dressing in colorful saris. In our boarding schools there is also a certain status associated with the event; one occasionally finds student leaders falsely entering their names in the book set apart for recording the dates of menstruation because they would feel insecure if other, younger, girls were to realize that they had not yet reached this particular stage of maturity.

The first menstruation may be expected between the ages of ten to seventeen—less than one in a hundred girls have not started by the age of sixteen years (Figure 16). If menstruation has not started, and providing that the girl is healthy in other respects, doctors prefer not to hasten the onset of menstruation before the age of eighteen years. Then, if menstruation does not start easily with a course of hormone therapy, full biochemical tests are advisable.

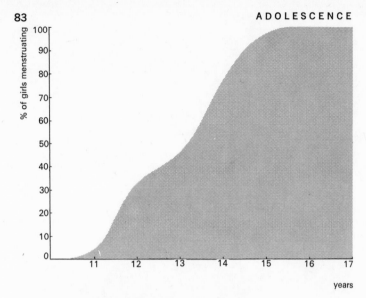

Figure 16. Onset of menstruation at puberty

Menstruation is not an isolated event. It is only part of a general growth into adulthood, which has already been proceeding for a couple of years. The earliest sign is usually the growth of axillary and pubic hair. Girls who look hopefully for a few isolated hairs under their arms seem not to realize that in a few years they will be spending as much time trying to remove these same offending hairs.

The next sign of growth is the very gradual development of the breasts. They do not grow overnight, but slowly develop from a small nodule beneath the nipples, at first merely the size of a grape, and then gradually spreading outward. Often one breast develops slightly before the other, but although this discrepancy is often so worrying that immediate medical advice is sought, it is nothing to be alarmed over. In due course both breasts develop, for the growth stimulus to the breasts comes from the pituitary gland which sends hormones in the bloodstream to stimulate the development of breast

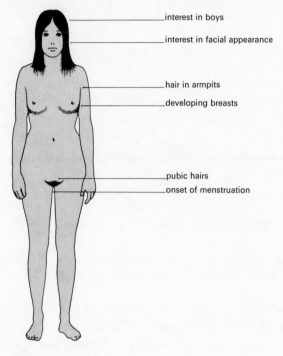

Figure 17. Secondary sex characteristics

tissue, and this continues until both breasts are fully formed (Figure 17).

The complete change from girlhood to adulthood takes about five years, with the onset of menstruation marking the halfway stage. Initially menstruation is not necessarily a regular monthly event. The first blood loss is likely to be followed by an interval of several months before the second menstruation, when there may be a further prolonged interval over the subsequent two years. One schoolgirl menstruated only at the beginning and end of each term for a couple of years and then gradually became regular.

The amount of blood lost during the early years is also variable. Sometimes there may be little more than a slight vaginal discharge, which gradually becomes red in color and increases in quantity. Those who start with such very slight monthly loss, gradually increasing in amount, are the ones most likely to develop a regular monthly pattern from the beginning. Other girls may have a full adult loss almost from the beginning. Some, while initially starting with a seven day loss, gradually find that over the next two or three years the duration of the loss settles down to the more usual four or five days.

With the first few menstruations ovulation does not usually occur. Although the lining of the womb is shed at intervals, there is no egg cell expelled from the ovary and therefore conception is not yet possible. The monthly spring-cleaning is occurring in preparation for the future. Spasmodic dysmenorrhea is unlikely to be found in the early years of menstruating life but comes with the occurrence of ovulation.

Sometimes, even before menstruation has started, the mother of an adolescent daughter may be aware of the monthly tantrums and sulks of her daughter. Teachers may recognize girls whose work shows marked variations, with excellent work one week but poor, untidy and careless work the following week. The girl herself will be finding it all very confusing and impossible to understand. The hormonal changes may be too much for her and she may have premenstrual tension even before menstruation has commenced. Cyclical patterns of misbehavior in girls who have not yet started menstruation are discussed in Chapter 23. Such children can still benefit from hormonal treatment, which is often required for a temporary period only.

The young child associates bleeding with cuts, falls, accidents, hurts and a multitude of painful experiences of the past. It is essential therefore that girls should know about the monthly blood loss before they reach puberty and experience it for themselves. The best course is to prepare the girl for the event and also to be ready to explain again and answer questions again as soon as the first menstruation has become a reality. Some authorities suggest that children should be told the facts of life as early as five years. Admittedly these children cannot appreciate the full significance of menstruation, but once the initial idea is implanted it can be built upon as the opportunity arises. In any case the teaching about menstruation and pregnancy should be gradual and not repetitive; interesting and not prolonged; preferably given when sought; and, ideally, undertaken by the mother. There are plenty of good books and pamphlets which the mother can use to help her find the best words for what she has to say and to ensure that the young girls in her charge are prepared for this event well in advance.

The changes of puberty are physiological, emotional and physical. It can all be most confusing to a girl, and she needs at this time, more than at any other, understanding, security, and love to see her through this changing pattern of life.

# 16

# Change of Life

When the years of childbearing are over the body reverts again to its girlhood pattern. The change of life is like the changes of adolescence in reverse. Puberty averages five years for its completion and so does the change of life. The amount of hormonal stimulations from the pituitary gland to the ovaries and the womb diminish. The ovaries stop producing their egg cells, the womb changes its endometrium less frequently and as the breasts are no longer required for breast feeding they also diminish in size. Although the pituitary stimulation is decreasing, the other glands often try to work overtime to compensate, bringing overactivity of the thyroid and adrenal glands.

It is only the faculty of childbearing which is lost at the change of life; the femininity, sexuality and attractiveness remain. To a woman in good health, physically and mentally, there is no reason any longer to fear what our grandmothers called "the difficult age." It is a time when there may be renewed vigor and when sex can be enjoyed without the ever-present fear of conception. The "Middle-age Spread" begins at this time, making the obese put on still more weight; and what is not generally appreciated is that at this time those who are too thin often lose weight and become even scraggier.

The last menstruation is termed the *menopause,* but one can never be sure if a given menstruation will be the last until at least two years have passed; therefore the exact date of the menopause can be timed only in retrospect. The medical word for the changes associated with cessation of the childbearing phases of life is the *climacteric.*

In Britain the average age for the menopause is between the forty-eighth and forty-ninth birthday, with an age range between forty and fifty-five years. Just as puberty is tending to occur earlier, so the menopause is coming later. Strangely enough it is usually just those women who started their first menstruations late, at sixteen or seventeen years, who are likely to finish first, while those who started early are also likely to continue menstruating well into their fifties. There is often a strong family pattern in the timing of the menopause, those whose mothers and elder sisters finished early are likely to finish early themselves, and vice versa. Sufferers from premenstrual tension tend to menstruate into their fifties, but, erroneously, they are inclined to blame the change of life for all their menstrual symptoms from the mid-thirties onwards.

Just as there is no ovulation for the first couple of years after the onset of menstruation so, during the last couple of years of a woman's menstruating life, ovulation is absent. Pregnancy is therefore rare in the change of life, or after there has been any alteration in the menstrual pattern; nevertheless it must always be suspected if there is a sudden cessation of menstruation during the forties.

There are three ways in which the change of life normally occurs: gradually; abruptly; and with an increasingly irregular menstrual pattern.

With a gradual ending, the loss becomes less each month for two or three years, the duration of menstrual bleeding decreases from perhaps five to two days and

89

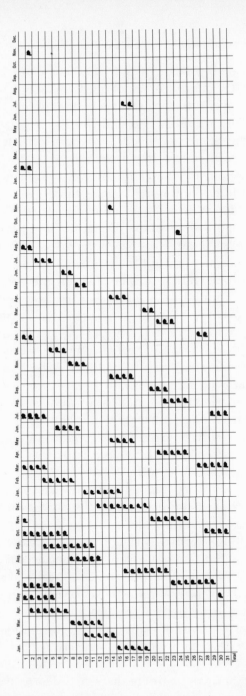

**P** = period

Figure 18. Gradual ending of menstruation at the menopause

then gradually menstruation becomes more irregular (Figure 18). If the dates of menstruation have been recorded over the years it becomes evident that the menstruation is not really haphazard in its irregularity, but still occurs at times it might have been expected. Thus if the normal cycle is four weeks, the intervals between menstruation may be eight, twelve, sixteen or twenty weeks, while if the usual cycle is three weeks the subsequent intervals will be multiples of three weeks. Women showing this type of menstrual pattern at the menopause will probably have a very trouble-free transition to their new era of life.

An abrupt ending of menstruation may occur if it coincides with a period of stress such as bereavement, moving to a new house or job, or children leaving home for marriage or college (Figure 19). This type is usually associated with fear of pregnancy but if one is able to inspect a menstrual record of these women, one often finds that over the previous two years there has been a gradual shortening of duration, so that while menstruation lasted six days during the childbearing years it may have diminished to three days before the abrupt ending. This type of ending is often associated with depression. Sometimes treatment of the depression causes the menstruation to restart, although with the shorter three-day pattern rather than the six days the patient might have experienced in her thirties.

Increasing irregularity can occur without any shortening in the duration of menstruation nor decrease in the amount of blood lost (Figure 20). Again, when one inspects the menstrual records over several years one can still recognize a cyclical pattern during the spells of irregularity in spite of many missed menstruations. With this type the final period may well last for a full seven or eight days.

Under normal conditions there should be no symptoms

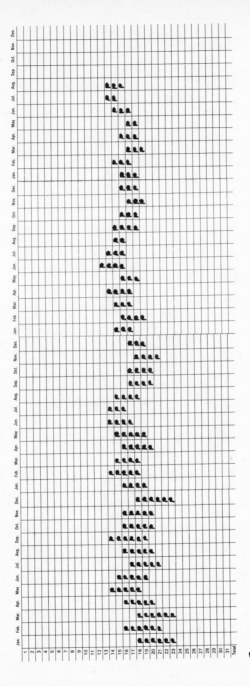

Figure 19. Abrupt ending of menstruation at the menopause

🦴 = period

92

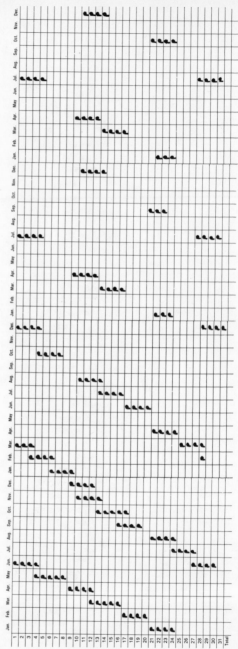

**P** = period

Figure 20.  Increasing irregularity of menstruation at the menopause

associated with the change of life, for this is a physiological process occurring gradually over several years. However, it is a time of many hormonal alterations in the pituitary, ovaries, womb, breasts, vagina, adrenals and hypothalamus, so occasional deviations from the normal are found. The commonest symptom and one which few women avoid, is the "hot flush." This is a sudden temporary flushing of the face and upper part of the body due to dilatation of the blood vessels. It lasts only a minute or two and may be accompanied by profuse sweating. It is caused by a temporary error of the thermostatic control due to diminishing and uneven hormonal output. Some women are acutely conscious of these flushes; they wrongly imagine that they are easily recognized by others, but this is probably true only where there is profuse sweating. Some women are satisfied with an open discussion about these curious and harmless sensations, while others come requesting treatment because they feel so self-conscious when working with men. Occasionally sleep is interrupted by the drenching sweats, which are so heavy that they disturb the husband's sleep. Women who suffer in this way, or from excessively frequent flushes, should receive treatment. The simple solution is a course of hormone tablets to correct the too rapid decrease in estrogen output.

Sufferers of premenstrual syndrome may well find their usual symptoms of headache, bloatedness, giddiness or tension present at the times of their missed menstruations as well as with the occasional menstruation (Figure 21). These cyclical symptoms may continue for about two years after the last menstruation, or until all the changes associated with the closing down of the menstrual clock are complete.

Women who have been given an artificial change of life by removal of the ovaries may suffer hot flushes immediately after the operation. It is interesting that, once

| | Jan. | Feb. | Mar. | Apr. | May | Jun. | Jul. | Aug. | Sep. | Oct. | Nov. | Dec. |
|---|---|---|---|---|---|---|---|---|---|---|---|---|
| 1 | | | | | | | | H | | | | |
| 2 | | | | | | | | H | | | | |
| 3 | | | | | | | H | | | | | |
| 4 | | | | | | | PH | | | | | |
| 5 | | | | | | | P | | | | | |
| 6 | | | | | | H | P | | | | | |
| 7 | | | | | | HP | P | | | | | |
| 8 | | | | | | HP | | | | | | |
| 9 | | | | | H | P | | | | | | |
| 10 | | | | H | H | P | | | | | | |
| 11 | | | | H | H | P | | | | | | |
| 12 | | | | H | | | | | | | | |
| 13 | | | H | P | | | | | | | | |
| 14 | | H | H | P | | | | | | | | |
| 15 | | P | | P | | | | | | | | |
| 16 | H | P | | P | | | | | | | | |
| 17 | | P | | P | | | | | | | | |
| 18 | | P | | | | | | | | | | |
| 19 | | | | | | | | | | | | |
| 20 | | | | | | | | | | | | |
| 21 | | | | | | | | | | | | |
| 22 | | | | | | | | | | | | |
| 23 | | | | | | | | | | | | |
| 24 | | | | | | | | | | | | |
| 25 | | | | | | | | | | | | |
| 26 | | | | | | | | | | | | |
| 27 | | | | | | | | | | | | |
| 28 | | | | | | | | | | | | |
| 29 | | | | | | | | | | | | |
| 30 | | | | | | | | | | | | |
| 31 | | | | | | | | | | | | |
| Total | | | | | | | | | | | | |

**P** = period    **H** = headache

Figure 21. Premenstrual headaches at times of missed menstruation

the other glands settle down again after the operation, the body reverts to its usual monthly rhythm, and every few weeks the woman may notice a temporary fullness of her breasts and a few days of tiredness. Those who previously suffered from premenstrual symptoms may find the usual symptoms recur at monthly intervals. The menstrual clock is situated at the base of the brain and this is not stopped merely by the removal of the ovaries or womb, but will be stopped only when the general reversal-changes marking the end of the childbearing era are completed. Should she have a recurrence of cyclical premenstrual symptoms these will still respond to treatment with progesterone.

If there has been an interval of two years since the last menstrual loss then any future bleeding should be viewed with suspicion and considered abnormal until proved otherwise. It is possible to have a really delayed menstruation after such a long interval of time, but on the other hand it may well be the first sign of excessively high blood pressure, of a growth or polyp or of some abnormality of the blood. The sooner any of these diseases are diagnosed and treated, the better. Every case of bleeding after an interval of two years is an indication that a thorough medical and gynecological examination is necessary, including inspection under an anesthetic of the neck of the womb, and also removal of scrapings of the endometrium for microscopic examination. With a markedly delayed menstruation it is usual to find that during the week or ten days prior to the bleeding the woman has suffered from all those symptoms which she normally associated with her premenstruum.

Already we have come to the end of a woman's menstruating life and as yet the effects of pregnancy have not been discussed. These are covered in the next chapter.

# 17

# The Effect
# of Pregnancy

Childbearing is the consummation of woman's biological function. All the changes that have taken place in her reproductive organs have been preparing her for it. The natural processes of generation seem to follow an uninterrupted rhythm in the whole of nature except for the human species. Already, in previous chapters, we have seen the difficulties which may arise in connection with the reproductive system of women; it would be surprising if these disturbances did not affect pregnancy and, in turn, pregnancy affect them. It is interesting to consider the effect of pregnancy on the two types of dysmenorrhea.

Already, the similarity that exists between premenstrual syndrome and toxemia of pregnancy has been mentioned. Toxemia heads the league of all known causes of death in childbirth for both the mother and the child, not only in Britain but in every country in the world. The treatment of toxemia that will be referred to, while not universally accepted, is highly successful.

When the fertilized egg cell beds itself down in the endometrium, a *placenta* (or afterbirth), is formed, interlocking with the endometrium for the nutrition and supply of the growth factors required by the developing fetus. As in the adrenals, so in the placenta: progesterone is formed as a halfway stage in the building up of most of the other placental hormones. The placenta begins forming at the moment of conception, but it does not become an appreciable hormone-production center until the fourth month, and from then onwards its production increases throughout the pregnancy.

Just before the baby is born, the placenta is producing at least a hundred times more progesterone than the non-pregnant woman produces when the normal level of progesterone is at its peak just before menstruation.

It is suggested that the new production center of progesterone in the placenta may produce:

1. The right amount of progesterone for the developing fetus.

2. Too much progesterone, in which case the mother will benefit by the excess.

3. Too little progesterone, in which case toxemia may develop.

Toxemia of pregnancy is characterized by the development in an otherwise healthy woman of high blood pressure, excessive weight gain, edema (extra fluid in the tissue), and passing of a protein (called albumin) in the urine. In severe cases the patient may develop fits, which are very harmful to both the mother and the child.

Examination of Figure 22 shows the effect of pregnancy on the three types of menstruation, premenstrual syndrome (including congestive dysmenorrhea), spasmodic dysmenorrhea and normal. During pregnancy when the placenta is producing an exceptionally high quantity of progesterone, sufficient for both the fetus and the mother, most sufferers from premenstrual syndrome benefit from the surplus of progesterone and experience excellent health, feeling "better than ever." They will be freed from their usual symptoms of headache, backache, depression, asthma or epilepsy, and find renewed energy. Some sufferers from premenstrual syndrome may find the

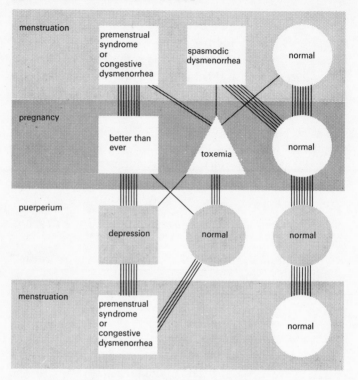

Figure 22. The effect of pregnancy on menstruation

placental production of progesterone insufficient for the baby's needs, and they will develop toxemia.

Most of the sufferers from spasmodic dysmenorrhea will have normal pregnancies, although there may be the unlucky few whose placental progesterone is insufficient and they too will develop toxemia. Again, most of the women who have trouble-free menstruations will also have trouble-free pregnancies, but the occasional woman will develop toxemia.

After the birth of the baby the placenta comes away from the womb, hence its name "afterbirth." The additional source of progesterone has therefore been removed. The time immediately following the baby's birth is called the *puerperium,* and during this time the woman's body adjusts to a normal progesterone level, which is a hundred times lower than the level she experienced during late pregnancy. This is responsible for the "puerperal blues" or tearfulness so frequent among women during those few days after the baby's birth. The woman, who previously suffered from premenstrual syndrome and who enjoyed such excellent health during pregnancy, may be upset by this sudden decrease in her progesterone level and may develop a more severe puerperal depression in which she becomes apathetic and tearful, losing appetite, interest, energy and initiative; she may also become sexually frigid.

When menstruation returns, perhaps three to nine months after the birth of the baby, those who previously suffered from spasmodic dysmenorrhea are likely to be free from further trouble. The body of the womb was stretched during the pregnancy and the neck of the womb was stretched by the delivery of the baby, so the periodic spasms of pain experienced when the menstrual blood forced its way through the neck of the womb are gone forever.

Those mothers who developed puerperal depression and those who had toxemia of pregnancy are, however, likely to have premenstrual syndrome when menstruation returns. About half the women suffering from premenstrual syndrome find it becomes more severe with each successive pregnancy. Fortunately progesterone treatment is still effective, in fact the woman who experienced "better than ever" health during pregnancy now knows the true feeling of "well-being" that can result when she receives sufficient progesterone.

The incidence of toxemia in different hospitals in England varies from 5 to 10 per cent, depending on such factors as prenatal care, proportion of first babies, of twins and the age of the mothers delivered in the hospital.

On a figure of five women in every hundred developing toxemia, three will previously have suffered from premenstrual syndrome, one from spasmodic dysmenorrhea and one will have experienced normal menstruation. However, nine out of ten women who develop toxemia of pregnancy subsequently suffer from premenstrual syndrome, and of those who have a second pregnancy also complicated by toxemia the incidence of subsequent premenstrual syndrome will rise to 100 per cent.

The exact cause of toxemia is unknown, although researchers all over the world are seeking for the answer.

A survey of 600 mothers attending the prenatal clinic at the Obstetric Hospital, University College Hospital, London, revealed that one in four of the expectant mothers who during the middle months of pregnancy felt ill with headaches, backaches, depression, giddiness and nausea, later developed toxemia of pregnancy. Whereas of the mothers who felt well during the middle months, only one in ten developed toxemia in the later months.

Progesterone was given to expectant mothers with toxemic *symptoms* (headaches, backache, depression, giddiness and nausea) in the middle months of pregnancy at the City of London Maternity Hospital and Chase Farm Hospital, Enfield. The results showed progesterone to be effective in preventing the development of toxemia, if given before the appearance of the *signs* of toxemia (raised blood pressure, edema, weight gain and albumin in the urine). But, once toxemic signs have developed, progesterone does not stop the steady deterioration of the patient's condition. The disease always ends once the baby and the placenta have been delivered.

There is abysmal ignorance about the metabolism of progesterone, but it is possible to hazard an explanation of the part progesterone plays in preventing, but not in curing, toxemia. If there is insufficient progesterone during the middle months of pregnancy three things occur, either in isolation or together: there might be the formation of abnormal harmful products from the faulty metabolism; there could be an excess of a certain corticosteroid, or there could be an insufficiency of a certain corticosteroid essential to the well-being of the pregnancy. Any of these occurrences could cause an accumulation of abnormal products capable of poisoning the mother, especially her kidneys, and causing the recognized signs of toxemia.

Progesterone for the prevention (as opposed to the cure) of toxemia has now been used for some fifteen years. Perhaps the most exciting outcome has been the appreciation that children born to mothers treated with progesterone appear to develop earlier and make excellent progress at school. A careful follow-up of children treated at the City of London Maternity Hospital between 1955 and 1957 has been made of each "progesterone" child (child whose mother received progesterone during pregnancy), now aged between nine and eleven years. Each progesterone child has been compared with the next child born to a healthy mother in the laborward register, and the next child whose mother developed toxemia. The head teachers of these children were asked whether the named child was "average," "above average" or "below average" in verbal reasoning, English, arithmetic, craftwork and physical education.

The results demonstrated that the progesterone children show a definite advantage over the control children in all the academic subjects. Further, the beneficial effects on these children appeared to be related to the dose of progesterone the mother received: the higher the dose the better the academic achievement. There is also a relationship between the time the progesterone was first given— the earlier in pregnancy the better the subsequent educational progress (Figure 23).

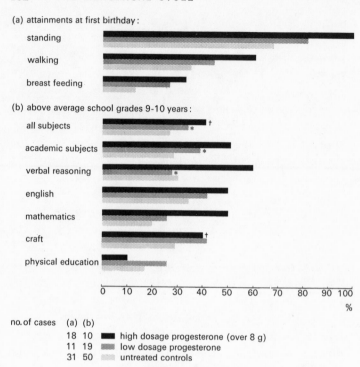

Figure 23. The effect of prenatal progesterone on intelligence

The children of the mothers who were treated with progesterone and of the control mothers who were chosen during pregnancy in the series at Chase Farm Hospital, Enfield, were examined by the medical officers or health visitors on their first birthday. It was found that progesterone children fared better—more were standing and more were walking at one year. Again the best results were from mothers who had received a high dose of progesterone during pregnancy.

This exciting news merely demonstrates how much more work there is left for our medical research workers to do. It may however give comfort to those who do require progesterone during pregnancy to know that it will do no harm to their unborn baby. Also a hormone which can be beneficial to an unborn babe is unlikely to be harmful to a non-pregnant woman even if used for long periods.

Up to now we have been concerned with the problems of being a woman, but when a woman is married there is another side to be considered—the effect of all this on the husband and children.

# 18

# The Menstrual
# Influence on Men

Unfortunately, the menstrual influence on a woman is not confined to herself. The effect spreads to those who are in close contact with her. It is difficult to make a statistical assessment of the full effect on the male, whether he is father, husband, fiancé or son. This chapter discusses a variety of situations in which the menstrual influence cannot be ignored.

Fortunate is the husband who is merely the onlooker when his wife has premenstrual tension; more commonly he is the butt of her irritability and depression. Women are always more likely to hit out at those nearest and dearest to them. One wrote, "Why am I always so unpleasant to my husband, and to a lesser degree my family, during the few days before menstruating? My behavior leaves everyone, including myself, completely bewildered —it is almost as though I become a totally different person. When my periods start I become normal again." Another pleads, "If only you could give me something so that I'm not so spiteful against my fiancé, whom I really do love."

Household worries that would be laughable at other times suddenly loom larger than life. A sharp word or a tactless remark can make the woman burst into helpless tears. One husband described how he knew by the way his wife woke up that he'd be able to do nothing right that day and that his loved wife would unaccountably lose her usual sense of humor and understanding and turn into a nagger. She would suddenly complain about things that had been going on happily all the month, like the way he read his paper at breakfast, his habit of slamming the door or the way he opened his letters; minor everyday events became a major source of irritation. Nor could he take her to a pub to ease the tension for during her premenstruum she became more sensitive to the effect of alcohol and one glass could easily have the effect of two.

When it gradually dawns on the husbands that there is a periodicity in their wives' personality changes, they are able to take steps to avoid obvious points of conflict. One husband asked the bank manager to send the monthly statement on the tenth day of each month, rather than the first day which was liable to become an extra source of tension for his wife. Instead they could now discuss their financial position in the calm of the intermenstruum.

Wise marriage guidance counselors are aware of the mischief that can arise from the premenstrual irritability and draw the attention of both members of the marriage to the way in which their quarreling is related to the menstrual cycle. One counselor arranges to see both partners eight days after they quarrel; in this way he hopes that the woman will have safely passed both her premenstruum and menstruation before the time of interview.

It is not necessarily the husband who suffers; it may well be the son who is influenced by his mother's cycles. A colleague studied the attendance records at a light-industrial firm for lateness and absenteeism among both men and women employees. She thought she had detected a tendency for a few of the men to have monthly spells of lateness, and it transpired that the men were late to work because the wife or mother had overslept or was slower than usual preparing the breakfast or sandwiches. When the men's lateness charts were compared with those of their womenfolk the menstrual influence was clearly seen.

When a woman, whether she is an adolescent or mother, drops a tray of tea cups, how much better to say light-heartedly, "Just the wrong day of the month," than remonstrate with her on her clumsiness. She herself would rather not be clumsy, irritable, impatient and bad-tempered, and she doesn't understand why she is like this. The lack of insight by a woman when she is in her premenstruum is surprising, for a few days later when the menstrual influence has passed she can understand it all completely.

Some years ago a forty-year-old chef was disabled with chronic bronchitis, which was complicated by periodic exacerbations during which he would have a rise of temperature and increase in bronchial spasm. Careful examination of his records showed him to be having attacks at four-weekly intervals. After the situation had been discussed with him, he was given a month's course of testosterone, the male hormone, but unfortunately with no response. He was then given a month's course of progesterone, but again with no improvement. Treatment was then continued on the more orthodox lines. About a year later his wife sought treatment for menstrual irregularity and was found to have a large ovarian cyst. At the operation both ovaries were found to be diseased and were removed. After this the chef continued to have his chronic bronchitis, but the monthly exacerbations disappeared, a convincing demonstration of the effect his wife's menstrual problems had had on his health.

Men often seek medical advice because of recurrent

attacks of migraine, asthma or giddiness. Nowadays the husband is likely to be given a chart on which to record the dates of his symptoms, and the wife is encouraged to cooperate and record her menstrual dates as well. The husband may receive symptomatic treatment for his symptoms, and if they are found to be occurring in relationship to his wife's menstruation she receives specific hormone treatment.

A door-to-door salesman asked for help. He worked on a commission basis and while his average takings were about $200 per week, in one week in every four the sum fell to something nearer $50. Not only did he find it difficult to plan to make ends meet financially, but he felt his chances of promotion were affected. He explained that he became more depressed and seemed to start work later during the weeks his earnings were low. When asked about his wife's menstruation he immediately appreciated the significance of the question. At his next visit he brought along his wife's menstrual record which confirmed this suggestion. Her irritability and lethargy were unknowingly hindering her husband. Fortunately this condition is amenable to treatment, and in this case the husband's full cooperation was assured.

Depression is one of the symptoms which makes a woman cold sexually. Those with premenstrual depression may be handicapped in this direction. This does not help the husband, who is already trying to cope with her irritability and apparent laziness. Fortunately once the menstrual hormones have been regularized she is more likely to enjoy the sexual side of marriage too.

More than one woman has expressed the wish that it was possible to induce menstrual periods, "just a few—for male doctors and husbands." However it is not only the husbands who are affected. Recently research has produced some remarkable evidence of the influence of a mother's menstruation upon her children.

# 19

# The Effect on the Child

Children find sudden changes in the behavior of their mothers particularly difficult to understand. A mother who is generally placid but becomes bad-tempered in her premenstruum, or a mother who enjoys long walks some days, but is too tired and sits on the park bench on other days is perplexing to children whose boundless energy continues undiminished day by day. This inconsistency of the mother may produce feelings of insecurity in the child which result in emotional disturbances. A vicious circle may develop in which the child's reactions of insecurity add to the mother's worries concerning her ability to rear her child, so increasing her stress and resulting in even greater premenstrual instability. Whenever the serenity of the home is affected by the mother's premenstrual syndrome, then full hormone treatment is indicated.

A London evening newspaper in October 1964 told of a young mother who had been beating her three-year-old daughter. In evidence the mother said, "I suffer from my nerves, at certain times of the month it is worse than others." The husband said, "She seems to be quite uncontrollable. I have restrained my wife physically." This young woman was unknown to the author, but there was a similar instance in a kind and motherly patient, who in a fit of temper struck her child, fracturing a bone in her leg. In her case these violent outbursts always occurred just before menstruation was due, and treatment of her premenstrual tension resulted in a happy and even-tempered mother.

Serious cases of premenstrual tension can result in temporary loss of self-control, and many result in gross acts of violence. What happens in the less serious cases? Does the child show any adverse reactions to his mother's premenstrual irritability, depression and lethargy?

The story of Keith illustrates this point. He was a healthy three-year-old, brought to the doctor's office by his elder brother with an ultimatum that "something must be done." It transpired that he had been suffering from a "cold" since an attack of mumps ten months earlier; during tea that day Keith had again sniffed loudly, when, in his brother's words "Mother really lost her temper and made me bring him here." Keith was healthy enough and unconcerned by the thick nasal mucus coming from his nostrils. It was Keith's first visit since having mumps. Next day his father confirmed that Keith had had an undue share of recurrent colds, which had not been continuous, but each time one cleared up there was a recurrence within a couple of weeks. Father agreed to bring Keith regularly each week until his present cold cleared, and to report the development of any new cold immediately, recording the onset and duration of the colds on a chart. The mother was aged thirty-five years, in good health with painless normal menstruation, although she did admit to being tired and bad-tempered sometimes. When the dates of Keith's subsequent colds and his mother's menstruations are superimposed, as in Figure 24, it becomes obvious that this boy was reacting in his own way to her changed personality during the premenstruum.

During the months from March to October 1965

| | Jan. | Feb. | Mar. | Apr. | May | Jun. | Jul. | Aug. | Sep. | Oct. | Nov. | Dec. |
|---|---|---|---|---|---|---|---|---|---|---|---|---|
| 1 | | | | | | | | | | | | |
| 2 | | | | | | | | | | | | |
| 3 | | | | | | | | | | | | |
| 4 | | | | | | | | | | | | |
| 5 | | | | | | | | | | | | |
| 6 | | | | X | | | | | | | | |
| 7 | | | | X | | | | | | | | |
| 8 | | | | X | | | | | | | | |
| 9 | | | | X | | | | | | | | |
| 10 | | | | X | | | | | | | | |
| 11 | | | | X | | | | | | | | |
| 12 | | | | X | | | | | | | | |
| 13 | X | | | X | | | | | | | | |
| 14 | X | | | | | | | | | | | |
| 15 | X | | | | | | | | | | | |
| 16 | X | | | | | | | | | | | |
| 17 | X | | | | | | | | | | | |
| 18 | X | | | | | | | | | | | |
| 19 | PX | | PX | | | | | | | | | |
| 20 | P | X | PX | | | | | | | | | |
| 21 | P | X | PX | | | | | | | | | |
| 22 | P | X | PX | X | | | | | | | | |
| 23 | P | X | PX | PX | | | | | | | | |
| 24 | P | PX | P | P | | | | | | | | |
| 25 | | PX | | P | | | | | | | | |
| 26 | | P | | P | | | | | | | | |
| 27 | | P | | | | | | | | | | |
| 28 | | P | | | | | | | | | | |
| 29 | | | | | | | | | | | | |
| 30 | | | | | | | | | | | | |
| 31 | | | | | | | | | | | | |
| Total | | | | | | | | | | | | |

P = mother's periods    X = keith's colds

Figure 24. Relationship of a child's colds to mother's menstruation

records were made of all children coming to the office with minor coughs and colds. Of ninety-one children who came, 53 per cent were brought by the mother while she was in the four days before or during menstruation (Figure 25). The figure shows the menstrual cycle divided

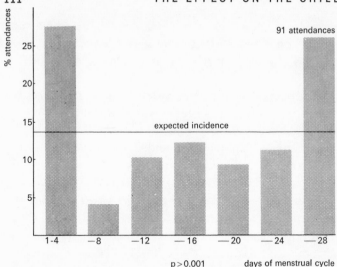

Figure 25. Doctor's office visits of mothers with sick children

into seven phases of four days each, on which an average distribution of 14 per cent for each four-day phase might be expected. However, in this survey there was a significantly high attendance of children with minor ills during mother's premenstruum or menstruation. The mothers most likely to attend with their children during the paramenstruum were those whose children were under two years, especially those with only one child, or those with children whose symptoms lasted less than twenty-four hours; and young mothers under thirty years.

A mother does not always take kindly to the suggestion that her child is being influenced by her changed personality at certain times of the month. Often it is easier to persuade her to be treated with a tranquilizing tablet rather than hormone treatment. If she is converted into a more placid and amiable mother, the child's asthma, cold or other symptoms will respond just as well. One mother who, when told of the possible relationship between her menstrual cycle and the child's ailments, said, "I remember with my elder son, whenever I had to sit up with him all night because of his constant cough, it always brought on my period." One wonders which came first.

An unexpected comment often heard after successful treatment of a mother's premenstrual syndrome is, "Even my children are more placid, they behave better."

A mother of two sons who tended to produce emotional colds whenever their mother menstruated has recently started training at a College of Education. She wrote: "I thought you would be interested to know that all the students who were practice teaching said that they had great difficulties with their classes when they were having periods—and so did I! It wasn't only that we were under par, but the children seemed to sense it, just as if we were their mothers!"

# 20

# The Effect
# on Schoolgirls

The hidden effects of menstruation and its impact, not only on the woman herself but also on others, have been demonstrated in previous chapters. It is now time to look at its influence on the adolescent as she goes through her school years.

In the studies of menstruation, adolescent schoolgirls form a useful sample population. Boarding schools have the advantage that the girls are removed from any adverse effects of their mothers' menstruation, such as have been described in Chapter 19, for the association with their schoolteachers is not so intimate, and is always more diffuse. Also, the groups of girls are all in the same age-range, and within each school the children are from similar social backgrounds. Many boarding schools take the routine precaution of asking the girls to record the dates of their menstruations. The wise matron will then scan the books occasionally to ensure that no girl is having excessively long or frequent menstruations. At one school the girls mail a card with their dates in a special box, so that girls cannot turn back the pages of the book to discover the menstrual pattern of other girls. The studies referred to in this chapter were made in four English boarding schools.

At one school the girls were given weekly grades, which

represented their marks for a given piece of homework in seven to twelve different subjects. Each weekly grade was compared with the grade obtained in the previous week to determine whether it was better, the same or worse, and also allocated to the phase of the menstrual cycle, before, during, immediately after or in the interval. Figure 26 shows the cumulative effect of menstruation

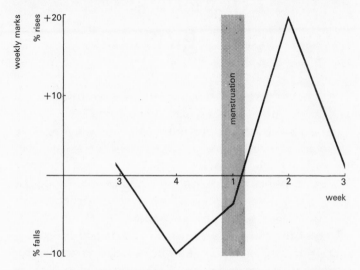

Figure 26. Variation in schoolgirls' weekly grades with menstruation

on 1,561 weekly grades. During the premenstruum there was a 10 per cent drop in working ability, with a commensurate rise of 20 per cent during the days immediately following menstruation. This is a wide fluctuation. One can almost hear the teacher saying to a girl, "Now I want you to try your very hardest this week and show me what you really can do." Unfortunately it is her premenstruum, so when the untidy and careless piece of work is returned, the comment is, "You could do better." The following week her work has improved and the teacher tells her, "Now if you really try you should be able to do a very good essay next week." Her menstruation is now over and her true ability is shown in her excellent essay. But all too soon another menstruation is due and her work again deteriorates. The girl's school report at the end of term most probably would read, "Mary can do good work when she tries." Would it not be fairer to say that Mary's work is severely influenced by her hormonal cycle?

More recently it has been possible to study the effect of menstruation on the results of various examinations. These showed that during the paramenstruum there were fewer passes, fewer honor grades and a lower average mark.

In the important "O-level" examinations, some subjects were completed on one day, some had papers within four days of each other, and some subjects had the individual papers eight or more days apart. Consideration of the results in relation to the time intervals between papers of the same subject showed that a girl was under a greater handicap in those subjects completed in one day, when she could be entirely in her premenstruum, compared with those subjects where the papers were spaced eight or more days apart. In the latter case a girl could not have been in the premenstruum and menstruation during both her papers. It should not be difficult for the various schools, examining boards and universities to appreciate the difficulties of girls taking examinations in their premenstruum, and so arrange the timetables that when a subject requires two or more papers these can be taken at an interval of a week or more apart.

When it is appreciated that a schoolgirl's entire future career may be determined by the results of public examinations, there would seem to be full justification for adjusting the menstrual cycle of those schoolgirls who know that they experience a phase of mental dullness during the premenstruum. Analysis of "O-level" results showed that it was those whose menstruation exceeded six days and whose cycle exceeded thirty days, who were most affected during the paramenstruum (Figures 27 and 28). Each individual needs to be considered separately for there are those on whom menstruation has no deleterious effect.

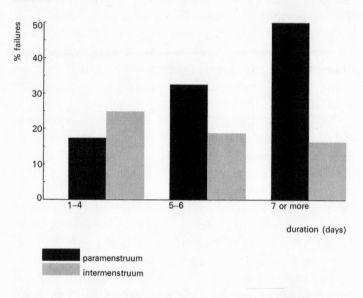

Figure 27. "O-level" failures and duration of menstruation

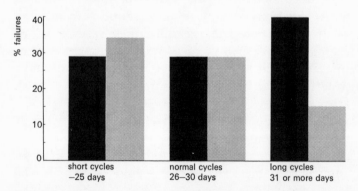

Figure 28. "O-level" failures and length of menstrual cycle

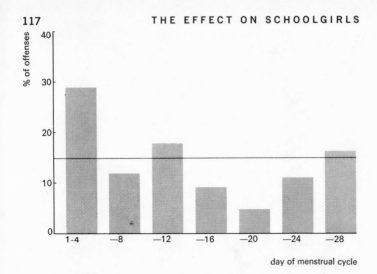

Figure 29. Schoolgirls' punishments during the menstrual cycle

At one school, punishment books were used for record-ing the names of girls, the date and the reasons for punish-ments. These books were made available for analysis. It was found that during menstruation the children were twice as naughty as might have been expected (Figure 29). Many of the punishments during menstruation were for offenses that could have been accounted for by lethargy, including forgetfulness and unpunctuality, and others were more probably a reflection on premenstrual irritability at having to conform to strict school dis-cipline. Indeed the girl with a slow reaction time during menstruation is more likely to be punished for any offense as she will be too slow to avoid detection. If several children are all talking when a teacher enters the classroom, it will only be those with a slow reaction time who will not stop talking quickly enough and will receive a punishment.

It was interesting to find that the "prefects," girls of sixteen to eighteen years, who were permitted to punish girls for misbehavior, gave significantly more punish-

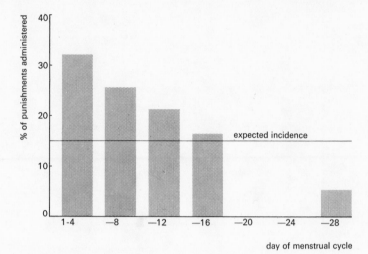

Figure 30. Punishments administered by prefects during their menstrual cycle

ments during their own menstruations and then gradually their standards fell throughout the cycle (Figure 30). This raises the important point as to whether the same is true of women generally, especially of teachers, magistrates and others in authority. Do they give more punishments during their own menstruation, and are they more severe? When they appreciate this possibility, will they lean over backwards to try and avoid punishing too severely when they themselves are menstruating?

One of my adolescent daughters burst into the house from school one day, asking for a menstrual chart. When asked why, she replied that her teacher had lost her temper and thrown a piece of chalk at a girl, and the same thing had occurred on the Thursday before half term, which was exactly four weeks earlier.

At another school, parents and visitors were invited to inspect the dormitories on the annual Open Day. There on the mantelpiece in each of the spotless dormitories was displayed a mark sheet, giving the marks each child

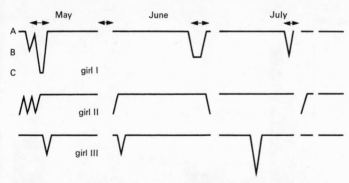

Figure 31. Schoolgirls' tidiness grades with cyclical drops

had received for the tidiness of her bed and locker before going down to breakfast each morning. It was not difficult on inspecting these sheets to determine the menstrual patterns of the girls, for when they were exceptionally sleepy during their premenstruum they were more likely to receive a poor tidiness grade (Figure 31).

There is a great need for teachers to appreciate the existence of premenstrual tension, recognizing that the girls in their charge may become irritable, disheartened or depressed at certain times, and they should be ready to step in with some encouragement, particularly in preventing a girl giving up a worthwhile career just because of some minor pin-pricks or temporary difficulties of study.

The code of behavior expected of schoolgirls appears to be far higher than for adults, who sometimes talk when requested not to in theaters and libraries, park where they are not allowed, and smoke when asked to abstain. Adults are not punished like schoolgirls, although they are often late for appointments. To compare the effect of menstruation on the behavior of adults in a closed community, studies were conducted in a women's prison. All newly convicted prisoners and all disorderly prisoners, who had been reported to the Prison Governor for misbehavior

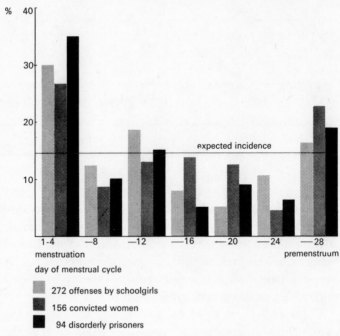

Figure 32. Times of schoolgirls' and women prisoners' offenses during the menstrual cycle

while in prison, were interviewed individually. The menstrual influence on the prisoners was the same as for schoolgirls (Figure 32) and half of all their crimes were committed either in the four days before, or during menstruation. This handicap of menstruation is similar for women of all ages, from the adolescent to the menopausal woman.

It seems probable that it was the slow reaction time that was also responsible for the punishment of many of the women prisoners, particularly in crimes like theft and shoplifting, where the women were not quick enough or did not give the precautionary glance over their shoulders before committing the crime. Premenstrual carelessness appeared responsible for the detection of embezzlement and fraud. It also raises the point that to treat habitual criminals suffering from premenstrual syndrome might merely make them better criminals and detection harder.

Crimes of violence by a woman, either against her husband, child or others, reflect woman's premenstrual irritability, and such crimes predominate in this phase of the cycle. A similar survey in New York revealed that 62 per cent of crimes of violence were committed during the premenstruum. The Parisian police records in the early part of the century showed that 84 per cent of crimes of violence committed by women occurred during the premenstruum or menstruation.

Alcoholics were often arrested during their premenstruum, possibly because when there is any significant degree of water retention the effect of alcohol is increased. One prisoner, with many previous convictions for drunkenness, confided that she always began to menstruate when in the cells of the local police station.

# 21

# Women
# at Work

British industry loses 120 million working days a year because of the menstrual problems of eight million women employees. Parker, in 1960, estimated the loss to industry in the United States as five billion dollars annually. These figures are astonishingly high, and too large to imagine in terms of individuals, but to a woman who feels she is alone in her misery it may help her to realize how worldwide the problem really is. The premenstrual syndrome has been described as the world's most common disease.

The menstrual influence on mental ability found in the schoolgirls also occurs throughout a woman's menstrual life, although in later years it is harder to obtain for analysis a sample population of women of the same age and doing the same work. One has only to watch typists in a large pool and notice how on one day some typists are filling their wastepaper baskets with spoiled work, and on other days it is a quite different group of typists doing the same thing. More than one understanding woman employer has asked for medical advice on behalf of a secretary whose mistakes reach unduly high figures during the premenstruum or menstruation.

The menstrual influence affects women in all grades and all skills of employment from the top executives who

make hasty decisions, errors of judgment or are temporarily deprived of drive and initiative, to the office assist-
ant who slops the coffee on the saucers with such
regularity. A wise admissions officer once said that he
knew when the local women doctors had their "off days"
as they would send patients into the hospital with less
discrimination. One of my cleaners always revealed her
premenstrual phase by leaving a can of Ajax on my
dressing table, or the carpet sweeper in the middle of
the living room.

Similarly the effects of menstruation are apparent in all
phases of woman's employment. A woman's success at her
initial interview may well result from the fact that she is
in her bright postmenstrual phase. But during employment there will be days when she is at the mercy of premenstrual forgetfulness, clumsiness, inattentiveness and
mental dullness. Finally she may lose her job because of
a sudden fit of premenstrual irritability, the irrationality
of her forewoman, her own unpunctuality or her regular
once-a-month absences. Analysis of her time sheet or
piecework earnings may reveal her menstrual pattern.

The particular handicap experienced by the individual will be more marked in certain employments than
others. Thus intermittent lack of manual dexterity particularly affects those workers with manual skills. One
chiropodist complains that during the premenstruum her
hands go stiff and she finds skilled movements difficult. "If
ever I do cut a patient you can be sure it's during those
premenstrual days." Those whose work depends on speed
and mental clarity, such as typists, are exposed to other
special difficulties, including clumsiness, lack of concentration and slow reaction time. On the other hand these
symptoms may not be so vital to shop assistants, who are
likely to be handicapped more by becoming irritable or
impatient with their customers.

The site of an individual's premenstrual symptoms

may be determined by her type of work. In 1954 an investigation into the incidence of premenstrual syndrome included a survey in a light-industrial factory employing some 3,000 women. These were interviewed separately in batches of about twenty per day. Some days it was noted that the predominant premenstrual symptom was backache, and on other days headache was not only the commonest symptom but present in most members of the batch. Later it transpired that all the women in any one batch came from the same department and were doing the same kind of work. Those who spent their working hours bending over a workbench were more likely to complain of premenstrual backache, while those employed sitting at a bench assembling minute electrical parts, a task needing considerable mental concentration, were mostly those complaining of premenstrual headache.

Employees in a light-industrial firm and also in a chain store revealed the familiar picture of half of all women reporting sick during or immediately before menstruation. Drs. W. Bickers and M. Woods in 1951 demonstrated that in an American industrial plant employing 1,500 women, 36 per cent of the women requested sedation during the premenstrual week. Dr. Robert Goldblatt of Georgia estimated that in 1955 premenstrual tension cost the state nearly three weeks a year per female employee in absence or reduced efficiency.

Accident proneness, which is discussed fully in the next chapter, is another handicap. The findings were confirmed by a survey of accidents among 10,000 women industrial workers in the Midlands, in which it was found that accidents were especially common during the premenstruum and menstruation. Mr. Norman Capener, scientific director of the Medical Commission on Accident Prevention, has even suggested that this accident proneness would be reduced if there were more widespread use of the contraceptive pill.

Some women discussed their difficulties when driving during menstruation. One tried to avoid driving as she tended to burst into tears each time the traffic lights were against her. Another confessed to having an almost uncontrollable urge to drive head-on at any oncoming car. A mother who daily drove her two sons to school gave them instructions on certain days that talking was forbidden, as she felt she could not adequately concentrate on driving during menstruation with all their chatter going on.

In Indonesia the fortunate women employees may take two days off each month under Trade Union Agreements. Some film stars have a clause in their contracts prohibiting close-up filming during menstruation or the premenstruum, when the puffy skin or dark rings under their eyes might not be flattering to their image.

Fortunately an increasing number of larger industrial organizations are supplying luxurious rest rooms for women. While these are highly desirable, one wishes that instead their industrial medical advisers would sift out those employees to whom a new lease of life could be given by the correct administration of hormone therapy and arrange for them to receive treatment. There is, however, the exceptional woman who does not wish for relief of her monthly incapacity. One example occurred when the author visited a teenager with flu in a slum dwelling. During examination her mother mentioned that her daughter was brought home from her West End office each month with period pains. They were reminded that nowadays such suffering was no longer necessary. The girl could hardly wait for the thermometer to be removed from her mouth before exclaiming, "Oh don't! How else could I get a ride in a taxi once a month?"

# 22

# Accidents
# or Coincidents

An important aspect of the hidden influences of menstruation is revealed in recent studies into hospital admissions. In 1959 it was shown that half of the women admitted to mental hospitals for acute psychiatric illnesses were either menstruating or about to begin. It might have been expected that the admission rate would be high for those with depression (47 per cent) and those who had made an unsuccessful suicide attempt (53 per cent), but it was surprising that the high figure persisted for other psychiatric illnesses like schizophenia (47 per cent), alcoholism, neuroses and the various organic psychoses. An added importance of these findings was that, by knowing the exact time in the patient's menstrual cycle, one could predict how soon recovery might be expected. A woman admitted four days before menstruation might be expected to deteriorate further until the onset of her menstruation, whereas another patient, just as ill on admission, who was already menstruating could be expected to improve within the next day or two. The added burden of menstruation appeared to work as a trigger factor on patients already mentally ill.

The high figures for attempted suicides during the premenstruum has been confirmed by Drs. A. J. and Mary P. Mandell on the Staff at the Los Angeles Suicide Pre-

126

vention Center. When receiving calls from women threatening to take their lives, they asked them about their menstrual dates. Half of the distressed women were expecting menstruation within a few days. Similar figures have been obtained by Drs. Pamela and the late I. L. MacKinnon when performing post-mortems in England, and also by Dr. A. L. Ribeiro working among Hindu women in India. The worldwide influence of premenstrual depression again becomes evident from these studies.

Later, a survey in the accident wards of four London hospitals revealed that half of all women involved in accidents were admitted to hospital in those vital paramenstrual days. Some admissions were the results of accidents at home, some on the road, some in factories, some women were passengers and some were drivers, but the influence of the paramenstruum was the same (Figure 33). It seems to be a slower reaction

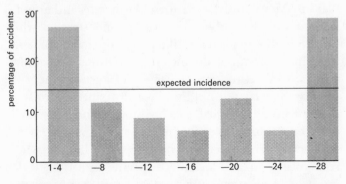

Figure 33. Accident admissions during the menstrual cycle

time which accounts for the injuries. Thus, in the short interval of a few seconds when a car mounts the curb and before hitting a brick wall there is just sufficient time for an alert passenger to brace herself and cover her head, while the woman with the slower reaction time is too dull to take these elementary precautions. There was a high incidence, too, among those doing routine everyday tasks, like walking up stairs, making tea and cooking, but it was only on those days when the woman was mentally dull with a slow reaction time that these everyday tasks became dangerous.

Tranquilizing drugs are often prescribed for women with premenstrual tension and irritability, but in view of these findings of accident proneness during and before menstruation it seems foolish to increase their mental dullness and further to slow their reaction time with such drugs.

It has also been shown that even in the case of acute medical emergencies, like coronary thrombosis or bronchitis, or the surgical emergencies like appendicitis, half of the women were in the premenstruum or were menstruating at the time of admission to hospital.

In the hospital for infectious diseases it became evident that infections caused by viruses, like measles and mumps, were admitted mostly during the premenstruum, while infections due to bacteria, like pneumonia and abscesses, were more frequent during menstruation. This difference may be because in the bacterial infections there are usually a few days of mild illness before the serious stage of the disease is reached, so admissions do not necessarily occur on the first day of the infection. On the other hand, the bacterial infections may have occurred in those whose resistance is already lowered by a viral infection, which occurred in the premenstruum. Pneumonia, for instance, often occurs in one already lowered by virus infection. The other possibility exists that the timing of acute stages of bacterial and viral infections is associated with the different levels of estrogen, progesterone and other adrenal hormones during the premenstruum and menstruation.

The importance of estrogen and progesterone levels

in altering the resistance to infections has been recognized by the veterinary profession. In 1953 Rowson and his colleagues demonstrated that womb infections in cows could be caused and controlled by varying the levels of estrogen and progesterone. Experiments showed that estrogens confer protection on rabbits against infection by pneumococci, on mice against streptococcal infections and on monkeys and mice against live polio vaccine.

Only the serious illnesses are admitted to hospital as emergencies; what of the milder illnesses? Analysis of workers at an engineering firm and at a chain store revealed that half of all female employees reporting to the sick bay were either menstruating or expecting to menstruate within a few days. It is interesting to note that even the vague diagnoses given by the nurses in these sick bays, without any further medical tests or examination, showed that infections due to a virus, e.g. common cold, occurred during the premenstruum, and bacterial infections such as sore throats and abscesses occurred during menstruation.

An explanation may be found here of the old wives' tale that taking a bath or washing hair during menstruation results in a "death of a cold." This may have arisen from the observation that pneumonia, bronchitis and the common cold are all more frequent during menstruation.

In general practice, half of the women under fifty-five who asked for a home visit, and who had a temperature over 100° F. were menstruating or expecting to begin menstruation within the next four days.

In Chapter 19 mention was made of the frequency with which mothers bring their children to the doctor when they themselves are in the lowest ebb because of menstruation. One mother came to the office four times during the eight-month survey, each time bringing a different combination of her three children. First she came with all three children, the following month with the eldest and youngest child, and on two subsequent visits she came with one child only. On each occasion the mother was in her paramenstruum and suffering from premenstrual lethargy, depression, irritability, abdominal bloatedness and painful breasts. She rejected any suggestion that she might be helped by treatment, and preferred a simple remedy for her children. The medicine bottle provided some positive reassurance that she had not neglected her children.

A survey, not yet complete, of the time children are admitted to hospital as an emergency also suggests that there is a relationship to the phase of the mother's menstrual cycle. A two-year-old fell and broke his leg on the wet kitchen floor, while his menstruating mother was busy scrubbing. Perhaps it was a coincidence, but if she had been more alert she might have warned the child about the possible danger, or her reaction time might have been quicker, and she would have caught the child before he fell.

Another child was admitted having been scalded with boiling water while mother was making tea. The mother was menstruating. The circumstances were similar to those in which adults were admitted with scalds during the paramenstruum. Perhaps it is just a matter of chance whether it is the child or the mother who is involved in such an accident.

Many of our children's admissions to hospitals today tend to be "social" ones, where the mother is worn-out caring for the sick child, who perhaps has a chronic ailment like asthma, spasticity or mental deficiency. The child is admitted to give mother a rest. Such admissions are arranged when the mother is at the end of her tether and probably during her paramenstruum.

To doctors in hospitals caring for the aged and chronically sick, the geriatric wards appear to be constantly filled. If one bed is emptied, a new arrival fills it within hours.

How can these admissions also be influenced by menstruation? To the family doctor the picture is clear. There are a number of elderly geriatric patients who are on the regular visiting list. Gradually, they get weaker, deteriorating week by week, slowly becoming more bedridden, while they are lovingly nursed by their daughter or daughter-in-law. Then suddenly—and it is always suddenly—the day comes when the amateur nurse can manage no longer. All the difficulties of the patient are related to the doctor in a more detailed and possibly more exaggerated manner than usual. "Something must be done," is the cry. Sometimes the husbands come to the doctor to add weight to the request for hospital admission. A discreet inquiry at this moment invariably reveals that the daughter, who has reached the end of her tether, is due to begin menstruating. The task suddenly assumes immense proportions and she can continue nursing her loved patient no longer. The next week she will probably say she's a new woman now that she is eased of her nursing burdens (or could it be that she is now in her postmenstruum?).

# 23

# No Evidence
# of Male Cycles

So the picture builds up of the impact of the various ramifications of menstruation on the individual and on society. The widely differing effects of menstruation have a remarkable similarity in frequency of occurrence during the paramenstruum. It has been shown that half of the women investigated were found to be in their paramenstruum in studies of:

1. Newly convicted prisoners.
2. Disorderly prisoners.
3. Schoolgirls punished for minor offenses at school.
4. Women asking for a home call.
5. Accident admissions.
6. Sufferers from acute mental disturbances.
7. Employees reporting sick.
8. Acute medical and surgical hospital admissions.
9. Viral and bacterial infections.
10. Mothers of sick children.

By now the reader may be wondering whether men are similarly affected by their own hormonal cycle.

To find the answer to this question an analysis was made of the time interval between two specific occurrences. This can be done without reference to menstrual dates and so can be done in respect of men as well as women. Among the school punishments it was noted how many children, having been punished on one day, would be punished again within four, eight, twelve or more days. During one term 221 girls who had already started menstruating, 186 girls whose menstruation had not yet started and 307 schoolboys, had been punished, and their record cards were available for study. In both sexes it was found that if a schoolchild was punished once, there was a strong possibility that he or she would again be pun-

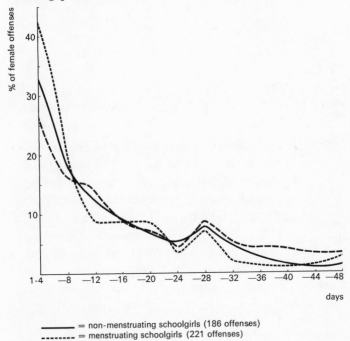

= non-menstruating schoolgirls (186 offenses)
= menstruating schoolgirls (221 offenses)
= female prisoners

Figure 34. Time interval of offenses committed by schoolgirls and female prisoners

ished within four days (Figures 34 and 35). If four days passed without a punishment their chances of another punishment were halved during days 5–8 after the first punishment. Again, if they succeeded in being good for

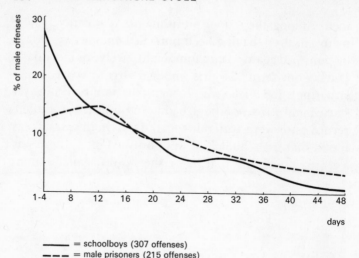

= schoolboys (307 offenses)
= male prisoners (215 offenses)

Figure 35. Time intervals of offenses committed by schoolboys and male prisoners

eight days their chances of misbehavior during days 9–12 were again decreased, and so on until by the 24th day when the chances for all groups were below 5 per cent. After that the difference in the sexes became evident for the girls showed a sudden rise in punishments between the 25th and 28th day, which was absent in the schoolboys.

A similiar analysis was then made in respect of male and female prisoners, who were reported to the Prison Governor for some offense while in prison. Both groups had a similar initial high recurrence rate during the first four days. This gradually dropped over the subsequent twenty days, but in the women between days 25 and 28 there was a secondary peak of offenses (Figures 34 and 35).

There is an eye condition, known as glaucoma, in which the pressure of the fluid within the eye is raised. Patients suffering from this condition may have periodic attacks of pain centered in the eye. In the women, over half of these attacks of pain occur during the paramenstruum, and it had been shown that the intra-ocular pressure, rise in blood pressure and body weight occur simultaneously with the pain in the eye. Both men and women can suffer from glaucoma, and patients under fifty-five years attending the Glaucoma Clinic at the Institute of Ophthalmology, London, were asked to record on a chart the times of attacks of eye pains. The results were analyzed for the interval between the first day of one attack and the same of the next attack. The same incidence of initial recurrence during the first four days was found in both sexes. Thereafter, the longer patients were without an attack, the better their chances of not having another. However between days 25 and 28 after an attack the women showed a secondary peak in the recurrence rate (Figure 36). This figure for intervals between attacks

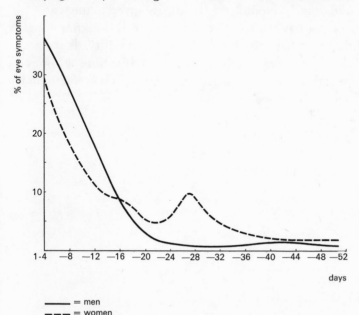

Figure 36. Time interval between attacks in patients with glaucoma

of glaucoma is remarkably similar to the intervals between punishments of schoolchildren and the punishments of prisoners by the Prison Governors.

This would suggest that if men do have hormonal cycles they are not associated with periods of indiscipline or lowered pain threshold, rise in intra-ocular pressure or blood pressure. Alternatively the findings could be interpreted as showing that the length of any male cycle must be so irregular as to be imperceptible in an analysis of this type.

In examples already mentioned where men have been found to have cyclical events (Chapter 18), such as the man with a monthly drop in his commission rate, men with cyclical lateness to work or with recurrent attacks of asthma, they have all, on more careful examination, been found to be related to the wife's menstrual cycle, and as such responded to treatment given to the wife.

In our present state of knowledge it does not appear that men have rhythmic cycles of irritability, depression, mental or physical lethargy, slow reaction time or lowered pain threshold such as occur in women in relation to their menstrual cycles.

# 24

# Conclusion

While reading this book some women will no doubt have recognized themselves with their personal idiosyncrasies. Others, who are blissfully free from menstrual problems, may suddenly understand some previously unexplained action of another woman. Male readers will have found a new understanding of the women around them, their peculiarities and the extent to which they are at the mercy of their menstrual cycles.

The need to understand women is of outstanding importance in some professions, such as those of magistrate, teacher, social worker, marriage guidance counselor and forewoman, but the social responsibility of greater understanding belongs to everyone.

Primitive society with its many taboos had the virtue that men recognized when women were menstruating. The idea of women going into purdah during those days has much to recommend it, but one does wonder what would be the effect on the national productivity if eight million women employees opted out for a few days each month.

There is much that women can do to help themselves. They can plan their engagements so that those days when they are most at risk are easier and they can get off to bed early and have plenty of rest. They can allocate their work, not undertaking an equal amount each day, but filling up the days early in the cycle so that there can be a more restful time as menstruation approaches. They can try—although it is almost impossible—to control their tongues and their actions when they are bursting with anger and irritability.

Today when so much of the work in hospitals is achieved by working in teams, it would seem a logical development for a Dysmenorrhea Team to run a Dysmenorrhea Clinic, or would this be regarded as too insignificant? It would need to be manned by a gynecologist and an endocrinologist and to have the assistance of a general physician and psychiatrist.

Neglect of menstrual pain and premenstrual tension is responsible for untold suffering and unhappiness. The ramifications are of considerable national, social and personal importance. The need for further research is obvious, and if this book has done anything towards opening the eyes of medical colleagues as well as laymen to the vicissitudes of being a woman, the time spent on its preparation will have been well worthwhile.

# References

*page* 30 Sir James Frazer, *The Golden Bough,* Abridged Edition (New York & London, Macmillan, 1924).

*page* 43 N. Kessel and A. Coppen, *Lancet* (1963), 2, 61.

*page* 49 Erna Wright, *Painless Menstrual Periods* (New York, Hart, 1966).

*page* 54 H. E. Billig, *International Record of Medicine* (1953), 11, 166, 487.

*page* 54 Oleck, *International Record of Medicine* (1953), 11, 166, 498 (after "temporary insanity" on p. 54).

*page* 57 W. A. Thomas, *Journal of the American Medical Association* (1933), 101, 1126.

*page* 57 E. Novak and E. K. Novak, *Textbook of Gynaecology* (London, 1952).

*page* 80 Anne Hamilton, *Medical News* (1967), 10/13/67.

*page* 121 W. R. Cooke, *American Journal of Obstetrics & Gynecology* (1945), 49, 357 (at end of first paragraph, page 121).

*page* 122 A. S. Parker, *Medical Clinics of North America* (1960), 44, 339.

*page* 124 W. Bickers and M. Woods, *Texas Reports on Biology and Medicine* (1951), 9, 406.

*page* 124 N. Capener, *Birmingham Post* (1966), 5/14/66.

*page* 126 A. J. Mandell and M. P. Mandell, *Journal of the American Medical Association* (1967), 200, 9, 792.

*page* 127 P. C. B. MacKinnon and I. L. MacKinnon, *British Medical Journal* (1956), 1, 555.

*page* 127 A. L. Ribeiro, *British Medical Journal* (1962), 1, 640.

*page* 129 L. E. A. Rowson, G. E. Lamming, and R. M. Fry, *Veterinary Record* (1953), 65, 335.

# Glossary

*Adrenal glands* two glands situated above the kidney and responsible for producing numerous hormones.

*Aldosterone* hormone produced by the adrenal cortex for the regulation of water and salt balance.

*Anabolic* building up.

*Cervical smear* test for the diagnosis of cancer of the neck of the womb.

*Cervix* neck of the womb.

*Climacteric* change of life.

*Corticosteroids* hormones produced by the cortex of the adrenal glands.

*Diuretics* drugs capable of increasing the amount of urine passed.

*Dysmenorrhea* pain with menstruation.

*Endometrium* inner lining of the womb.

*Estrogen* hormone released from the ovary.

*Fallopian tubes* two tubes leading from the ovaries to the womb, along which the egg cells pass.

*Geriatrics* care of the elderly.

*Glaucoma* disease of the eye characterized by raised pressure in the eyeball.

*Gynecology* study of the diseases of the woman.

*Hormones* chemicals, produced by glands, which pass in the bloodstream to exert an action at a distant site.

*Hymen* thin membrane partially closing the entrance to the vagina in a virgin.

*Hypothalamus* specialized part of the base of the brain concerned with control of metabolism.

*Implant* pellets of drugs inserted into the tissue.

*Intermenstruum* part of the menstrual cycle not covered by the premenstruum or menstruation, usually days 5 to 24.

*Intra-uterine device* small contraceptive appliance inserted into the womb.

*Menopause* last menstruation marking the end of the child-bearing era.

*Menstrual clock* the specialized portion of the brain responsible for the cyclical timing of menstruation.

*Menstrual cycle* time from the first day of menstruation to the first day of the next menstruation.

*Menstrual loss* bleeding at menstruation.

*Menstruation* monthly bleeding from the vagina in women of childbearing age, caused by the disintegration of the lining of the womb.

*Metabolism* building up and breaking down of chemicals in the body.

*Mittelschmerz* abdominal pain at the time of ovulation (middle pain).

*Ovary* reproductive organ containing the egg cells.

*Ovum* egg cell.

*Ovulation* release of the egg cell from the ovary.

*Paramenstruum* premenstruum and menstruation.

*Pituitary* gland situated at the base of the brain and controlling many other glands.

*Postmenstruum* the phase immediately after menstruation.

*Premenstruum* the four days before the onset of menstruation.

*Progesterone* hormone produced by the ovary for the preparation of the lining of the womb. Also a starting point for the production of numerous corticosteroids.

*Progestogen* synthetic preparation which builds up the lining of the womb in the same way as progesterone, but cannot be used for synthesis of corticosteroids.

*Spasmodic dysmenorrhea* spasms of pain occurring with menstruation.

*Syndrome* collection of symptoms which commonly occur together.

*Testosterone* male hormone.

*Therapy* treatment.

*Vagina* passage leading from exterior of the body to the mouth of the womb.

# Other publications
# by Katharina Dalton

THE PREMENSTRUAL SYNDROME. Joint authorship with R. Greene (1953), *British Medical Journal,* 1, 1007.

SIMILARITY OF SYMPTOMATOLOGY OF PREMENSTRUAL SYNDROME AND TOXAEMIA OF PREGNANCY AND THEIR RESPONSE TO PROGESTERONE (Charles Oliver Hawthorne B.M.A. Prize Essay– 1954), *ibid.,* 2, 1071.

THE PREMENSTRUAL SYNDROME (1955), *Proceedings of the Royal Society of Medicine,* 48, 5, 337.

THE AFTERMATH OF HYSTERECTOMY AND OOPHORECTOMY (1957), *ibid.,* 50, 6, 415.

TOXAEMIA OF PREGNANCY TREATED WITH PROGESTERONE DURING THE SYMPTOMATIC STAGE (1957), *British Medical Journal,* 2, 378.

MENSTRUATION AND ACUTE PSYCHIATRIC ILLNESSES (1959), *ibid.,* 1, 148.

COMPARATIVE TRIALS OF NEW ORAL PROGESTOGENIC COMPOUNDS IN THE TREATMENT OF THE PREMENSTRUAL SYNDROME (1959), *ibid.,* 2, 1307.

EFFECT OF MENSTRUATION ON SCHOOLGIRLS' WEEKLY WORK (1960), *ibid.,* 1, 326.

SCHOOLGIRLS' BEHAVIOUR AND MENSTRUATION (1960), *ibid.,* 2, 1647.

MENSTRUATION AND ACCIDENTS (1960), *ibid.,* 2, 1425.

EARLY SYMPTOMS OF PRE-ECLAMPTIC TOXAEMIA (1960), *Lancet,* 1, 198.

MENSTRUATION AND CRIME (1961), *British Medical Journal,* 2, 1752.

CONTROLLED TRIALS IN THE PROPHYLACTIC VALUE OF PROGESTERONE IN THE TREATMENT OF PRE-ECLAMPTIC TOXAEMIA (1962), *Journal of Obstetrics and Gynaecology of the British Commonwealth,* 69, 3.

THE PRESENT POSITION OF PROGESTATIONAL STEROIDS IN THE TREATMENT OF PREMENSTRUAL SYNDROME (1963), *Medical Woman's Federation,* July, 137.

THE INFLUENCE OF MENSTRUATION ON HEALTH AND DISEASE (1964), *Proceedings of the Royal Society of Medicine,* 57, 4, 262.

THE PREMENSTRUAL SYNDROME (1964), William Heinemann Medical Books, London.

THE INFLUENCE OF MOTHER'S MENSTRUATION ON HER CHILD (Charles Oliver Hawthorne, B.M.A. Prize Essay–1966), *Proceedings of the Royal Society of Medicine,* 59, 10, 1014.

THE INFLUENCE OF MENSTRUATION ON GLAUCOMA (Charles Oliver Hawthorne, B.M.A. Prize Essay–1967), *British Journal of Ophthalmology,* 51, 10, 692.

ANTE-NATAL PROGESTERONE AND INTELLIGENCE (1968), *British Journal of Psychiatry,* 516, 114, 1377.

MENSTRUATION AND EXAMINATIONS (1968), *Lancet,* 11, 1386.

THE ESSENTIALS OF CHIROPODY FOR STUDENTS (1938), Faber & Faber, London. Sixth edition (1968).

CHILDREN'S HOSPITAL ADMISSIONS AND MOTHER'S MENSTRUATION (1970), *British Medical Journal,* 2, 27–28.

# Index

*Numbers in italics refer to pages on which illustrations appear.*